Essentials of Respiratory Medicine

J.F. CADE MD, PhD, FRACP, FCCP
Director of Intensive Care,
Royal Melbourne Hospital, Australia

M.C.F. PAIN MD, FRACP, FCCP
Director of Thoracic Medicine,
Royal Melbourne Hospital, Australia

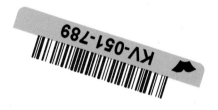

Blackwell Scientific Publications
OXFORD LONDON EDINBURGH
BOSTON PALO ALTO MELBOURNE

To our mentors,
Moran Campbell and John Read

© 1988 by
Blackwell Scientific Publications
Editorial offices:
Osney Mead, Oxford OX2 0EL
  (*Orders*: Tel. 0865-240201)
8 John Street, London WC1N 2ES
23 Ainslie Place, Edinburgh EH3 6AJ
Three Cambridge Center, Suite 208,
  Cambridge MA 02142, USA
667 Lytton Avenue, Palo Alto, California
  94301, USA
107 Barry Street, Carlton, Victoria 3053,
  Australia

First published 1988

Set by Setrite Typesetters Ltd Hong Kong
Printed and bound in Great Britain

DISTRIBUTORS
USA
  Year Book Medical Publishers
  200 North LaSalle Street
  Chicago, Illinois 60601
  (*Orders*: Tel. 312-726-9733)

Canada
  The C.V. Mosby Company
  5240 Finch Avenue East
  Scarborough, Ontario
  (*Orders*: Tel. 416-298-1588)

Australia
  Blackwell Scientific Publications
  (Australia) Pty Ltd
  107 Barry Street
  Carlton, Victoria 3053
  (*Orders*: Tel. 03-347-0300)

British Library
Cataloguing in Publication Data
Cade, J.F.
  Essentials of respiratory medicine.
  1. Respiratory organs — Diseases
  I. Title   II. Pain, M.C.F.
  616.2   RC731

ISBN 0-632-01913-1

Contents

Preface

Respiratory medicine has shared with other branches of medicine the many recent advances in laboratory and clinical medicine which have been based on new scientific knowledge and technological expertise. These advances have led not only to increased understanding of the mechanisms and processes of disease but also to changes in many practical aspects of investigation and treatment. It should be emphasized, however, that the fundamental value of previous major contributions remains and that the knowledge, particularly of physiology, acquired over the past 60 years continues to form the basis of respiratory medicine. This book thus attempts to summarize traditional teaching as well as to incorporate appropriate recent advances.

The purpose of this book is similar to that of others in the 'Essentials' series. It is to encompass in a small volume the essence of the specialty in a form suitable primarily for undergraduate medical students. However, it is hoped that the book could also be of use to general physicians, as well as to laboratory technologists, respiratory therapists and postgraduate nurses. A reading list has been appended for those wishing to explore individual topics in greater detail than is possible in a book of this size.

Many friends and colleagues have helped with various aspects of this book, although, as is customary, the authors retain responsibility for any errors or imperfections. Dr Jonathan Burdon, Professor Richard Larkins and Dr Paul Zimmerman each kindly reviewed the entire manuscript and their expert comments and suggestions are gratefully acknowledged. Professor Robert Clancy read the chapter on immunology and Dr Malcolm McDonald the chapter on respiratory infections, and their constructive criticisms are also acknowledged with thanks. Miss Kate Pain was responsible for drawing all the figures and we are grateful to her for her skilled assistance. We also thank Dr John Wilson for proof-reading the final manuscript, Miss Carmen Salerno for her patience in typing the many drafts required and Mr Mark Robertson of Blackwell Scientific Publications (Australia) for his unobtrusive support and liaison with the publishers. Blackwell Scientific Publications and Williams & Wilkins have kindly given permission for several previously published illustrations to be used as a basis for some of the figures in this book and the specific figures are so indicated in the text. Finally, we especially thank our families for their forbearance with ruined vacations and social disruption during the past year.

J.F. Cade, M.C.F. Pain
Melbourne

1   Structure of the Respiratory System

Structure-function relations

In many ways, the structure of the lung explains its function most elegantly. This is well illustrated by the anatomy of the airways in relation to ventilation, the blood vessels in relation to blood flow, and the blood—gas interface in relation to gas exchange. However, anatomy can be difficult to study in the live patient, and autopsy material often correlates poorly with the clinical and physiological derangements during life. Furthermore, many respiratory disorders comprise mixed disease forms or display considerable inhomogeneity, making anatomical correlation very difficult and usually quite imperfect in these circumstances.

Despite these limitations, knowledge of the structure of the respiratory system is important, not only for any correlation it may have with function, but also in its own right. Thus, structural considerations are integral to the understanding of many current diagnostic procedures, disease states and treatment modalities. For example, knowledge of the structure of the airways is important for the understanding of the findings at bronchoscopy, of the pulmonary vessels for the interpretation of pulmonary angiography, of the chest wall for the assessment of the consequences of trauma, and of the respiratory muscles for many of the aspects of mechanical ventilation.

Conducting airways

Much of the length, though not of the volume, of the respiratory tract comprises those parts which conduct gas (i.e. the tracheobronchial tree), as opposed to the gas exchanging areas of the lung (i.e. the alveoli). The conducting airways in turn are arbitrarily divided at the level of the cricoid cartilage in the larynx into the upper respiratory tract and the lower respiratory tract.

One of the chief additional functions of the upper respiratory tract (the nose, mouth, pharynx and larynx) is to filter, humidify and warm (i.e. 'condition') the inspired gas. The larynx also provides a means of controlling airflow, thereby protecting the lower respiratory tract against inspiration of noxious substances and modulating flow during expiration to permit speaking and effective coughing. The upper respiratory tract is responsible for about half of the anatomical deadspace and half of the resistance of the total respiratory tract.

The lower respiratory tract consists of multiple generations of branching airways which progressively decrease in diameter but increase in number and eventually in total cross-sectional area (Fig. 1.1). The dimensions of the branches and the angles of branching are close to those predicted on theoretical grounds to minimize the volume and resistance of the conducting pathway. There are 15–25 divisions or generations of airways depending on the site within the lung and thus the length of the pathway involved.

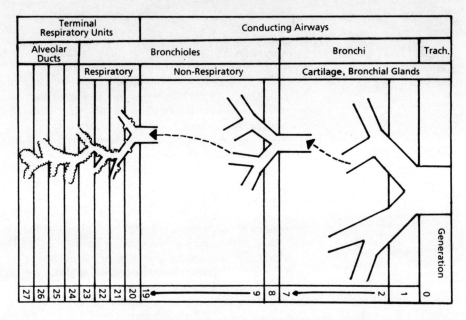

Fig. 1.1. Terminology of lung constituents showing a representation of airway subdivision down to alveolar ducts (redrawn from Crofton & Douglas, 1981).

The trachea divides in turn into two main (right and left), five lobar and 18 named segmental bronchi. The five lobes (three right, two left) are therefore divided into 18 broncho-pulmonary segments (ten right, eight left), corresponding to the segmental bronchi (Fig. 1.2). Although the fibrous septa between individual segments are incomplete, segmental anatomy is of importance in diagnosis and treatment of localized disease processes.

The segmental bronchi divide into subsegmental bronchi which are usually not specifically named. The small bronchi continue to divide until they are about 1mm in diameter, where cartilage is no longer contained in their walls and they are termed bronchioles. Bronchioles then divide into the terminal bronchioles, which are the final purely conducting airways. The physiologist's term 'small airway' refers to those structures less than 2 mm in diameter.

Right   Left

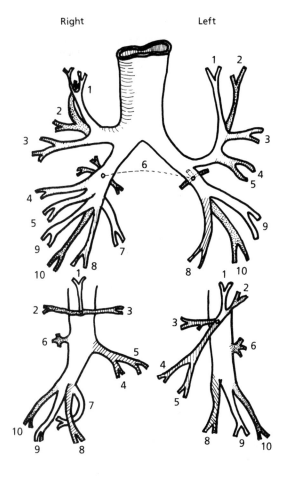

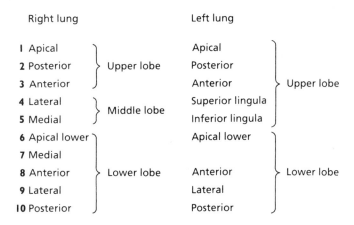

Right lung		Left lung	
1 Apical	⎫	Apical	⎫
2 Posterior	⎬ Upper lobe	Posterior	⎪
3 Anterior	⎭	Anterior	⎬ Upper lobe
4 Lateral	⎫ Middle lobe	Superior lingula	⎪
5 Medial	⎭	Inferior lingula	⎭
6 Apical lower	⎫	Apical lower	⎫
7 Medial	⎪		⎪
8 Anterior	⎬ Lower lobe	Anterior	⎬ Lower lobe
9 Lateral	⎪	Lateral	⎪
10 Posterior	⎭	Posterior	⎭

Fig. 1.2a. The bronchial tree as far as the segmental bronchi with anterior view above and lateral view below (modified from Crofton & Douglas, 1981).

3/*Structure of the Respiratory System*

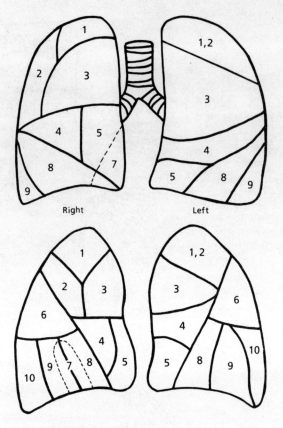

Fig. 1.2b. The surface anatomy of the bronchopulmonary segments with anterior view above and lateral view below (modified from Crofton & Douglas, 1981).

Gas exchanging units

From each terminal bronchiole arise up to 50 respiratory bronchioles, so named because they may have alveoli arising directly from them. Respiratory bronchioles continue to branch into two to five further subdivisions, until they end in alveolar ducts from which arise the alveolar sacs and then most of the alveoli themselves. Alveoli are the final blind-ends of the respiratory tract.

Those parts of the respiratory tract distal to the terminal bronchiole and concerned with gas exchange are the terminal respiratory units, referred to collectively as lung parenchyma and sometimes individually as acini or primary lobules (Fig. 1.3). An acinus consists of the respiratory bronchioles, alveolar ducts, alveolar sacs and alveoli arising from a single terminal bronchiole. A primary lobule is defined as an individual alveolar duct and its distal structures. A secondary lobule is the smallest portion of lung parenchyma bounded, albeit incompletely, by connective tissue septa. Each secondary lobule consists of three to five terminal bronchioles and their distal structures (and thus three to five acini). A secondary lobule is a useful anatomical or descriptive, though not

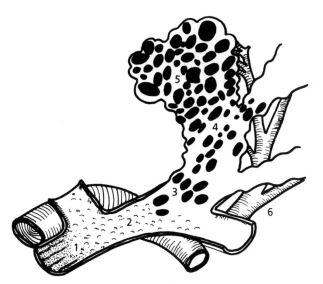

Fig. 1.3. Components of the lung acinus. (1) Bronchus. (2) Terminal bronchiole. (3) Respiratory bronchiole. (4) Alveolar duct. (5) Alveoli. (6) Pulmonary artery branch. (Redrawn from Nagaishi, 1972.)

physiological, entity in that it may be readily recognized macroscopically.

There are approximately 300 million alveoli in the average adult lung and each alveolus is about 250 μm in diameter. The total internal surface area of the lungs is thus extremely large, approximately 80 m². At birth, an infant has a full complement of airways but only about 25 million alveoli. Thus, although no new airways form after birth, most of the alveoli present in the adult have developed during childhood.

Communications between adjacent alveoli via pores of 10−15 μm in diameter permit gas flow between alveoli and segments of lung (collateral ventilation). These alveolar pores (pores of Kohn) may help prevent collapse when a local airway is occluded. Other alternative pathways for ventilation have also been described, such as the canals of Lambert which connect small bronchioles and nearby alveoli.

Histology

The structure of the airways changes progressively from the trachea to the alveoli. The mucosa of large airways consists largely of pseudostratified, ciliated, epithelial cells with deeper layers of cuboidal cells (Fig. 1.4). Scattered amongst the ciliated cells are mucus-secreting goblet cells. The number of layers of cells and the frequency of goblet cells decrease down to the terminal bronchiole. From the respiratory bronchiole, the airways are lined with cuboidal, non-ciliated, epithelial cells. The alveolar lining consists of two types of flattened, epithelial cells, type 1 and type 2 (Fig. 1.5). Most of the surface is covered with type 1 cells which by thin cytoplasmic extension constitute an important part of the blood−gas barrier. The more globular and granular type 2 cells are responsible for production and storage of surfactant. Scavenging cells such as macrophages also inhabit the alveolar spaces.

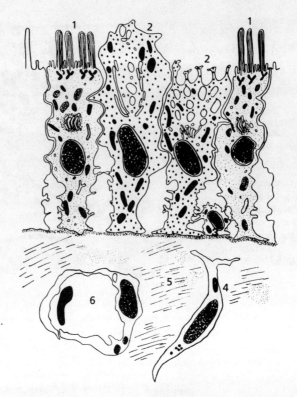

Fig. 1.4. Component structures in the bronchial lining. (1) Ciliated cell. (2) Goblet cell. (3) Basal cell. (4) Fibroblast. (5) Collagen fibres. (6) Capillary. (Redrawn from Nagaishi, 1972.)

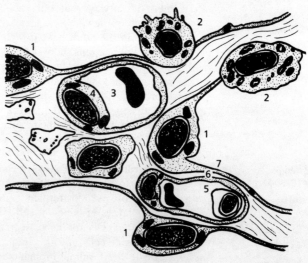

Fig. 1.5. Components of the alveoli. (1) Alveolar epithelial cell (type 1). (2) Alveolar epithelial cell (type 2). (3) Capillary with red blood cell. (4) Capillary endothelial cell. (5−7). The alveolar-capillary membrane — including contributions from cytoplasmic extensions of alveolar epithelial and capillary endothelial cells. (Redrawn from Nagaishi, 1972.)

Separated from the mucosa by the basement membrane is the submucosa. This contains an extensive capillary network, longitudinally arranged elastic fibres and mucous glands. The outermost part of the airway is the fibrocartilaginous layer. This contains cartilage, fibrous membrane and smooth muscle. Mucous glands and cartilage are found down to, but not including, the bronchioles (Fig. 1.6). Wisps of elastic fibres,

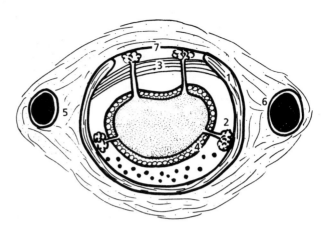

Fig. 1.6. A large bronchus in cross-section. (1) Cartilage. (2) Mucous gland. (3) Bronchial smooth muscle. (4) Mucosa. (5) Bronchial artery branch. (6) Pulmonary artery branch. (7) Fibrous membrane. (Redrawn from Crofton & Douglas, 1981.)

collagen and smooth muscle persist down to the alveolar walls. The fibrous support of the airways is connected to the surrounding peribronchial and septal connective tissue, forming a continuum of support throughout the lungs that is important in maintaining airway patency. As the horseshoe shape of the cartilage in the trachea and larger bronchi becomes more irregular in the smaller bronchi, the smooth muscle becomes more circumferential and is arranged in a spiral manner. Thus, it can shorten as well as constrict the airway.

The interalveolar septum comprises predominantly a capillary network between adjacent alveolar epithelial layers. Over much of the alveolar surface, the basement membranes of the capillary endothelium and alveolar epithelium are fused, so that the blood−gas barrier at this point is very thin (0.4−2.5 μm). Over the remainder of the alveolar surface, the two basement membranes are separated by the interstitial space, a thick part of the septum where fluid exchange takes place. The gas exchanging and fluid exchanging parts of the alveoli are thus anatomically separate.

Tracheobronchial secretions

The surface of the tracheobronchial tree is lined with a thin film of watery secretions. The goblet cells secrete mucus and the mucous glands secrete both mucus and serous fluid. Estimates of the total volume of bronchial secretions produced each day range from 10−100 ml. This biochemically complex fluid contains mucopolysaccharides and mucoproteins, and has both a sol and a gel phase. The sol phase bathes the cilia and a discontinuous gel phase lies on its surface. This blanket of fluid is conveyed proximally from the bronchioles to the larynx at a rate of 3−30 mm/min by ciliary motion. Normal ciliary function consists of a series of coordinated whiplike movements at a frequency of about 1200 beats/min in the sol layer. The mucociliary escalator is an important defence mechanism, particularly for the clearing of inhaled particles, which may be removed from the lung within hours. Many other substances are also secreted in the tracheobronchial fluid, including plasma proteins, immunoglobulins, antibodies, electrolytes and antibacterial substances such as lysozyme.

Surfactant

The gas exchanging areas of the lung are lined with a unique surface-active substance called surfactant. It is synthesized and stored in the alveolar type 2 cells and released as required onto the alveolar surface. It eventually denatures and is ingested by alveolar macrophages. Surfactant is a mixture of phospholipids, especially dipalmitoyl lecithin. By lowering the surface tension of the gas—fluid interface in the alveoli, it prevents alveolar collapse and permits much lower forces to expand the alveoli during inspiration than would otherwise be necessary.

Blood vessels

The pulmonary artery conveys virtually the whole cardiac output from the right ventricle to the alveolar-capillary bed. The pulmonary artery divides into right and left main arteries, which accompany and branch with the corresponding divisions of the tracheobronchial tree. As in the systemic circulation, the walls of large arteries (that run with the bronchi) are predominantly elastic and smaller arteries (that run with the bronchioles) predominantly muscular, but the thickness is much less because of the much lower intravascular pressures involved. The terminal arterioles which accompany the terminal bronchioles are end-arteries which supply the acini and break up into capillary networks in the alveolar septa. Although most of the pulmonary venous blood originates from the pulmonary capillary bed, some comes via direct arteriovenous anastomoses and some comes from bronchial veins in the walls of the larger airways and visceral pleura. Unlike the pulmonary arterial tree, the pulmonary veins drain into the interlobar septa and thus do not follow the tracheobronchial tree. They finally drain into the left atrium.

The lungs have a dual blood supply and receive blood from the bronchial arteries as well as from the pulmonary artery. The bronchial arteries are not constant in origin, arising generally from the thoracic aorta, but sometimes from the subclavian, internal mammary or intercostal arteries. They supply the bronchial wall as far as the terminal bronchioles.

Lymphatics

The lung substance as far as the alveoli is well supplied with lymphatics. These are situated in the peribronchial and perivascular tissues, in the bronchial walls and beneath the visceral pleura. Most alveoli have direct drainage via septal lymphatics but specific lymphatic capillaries do not exist in the actual alveolar-capillary space. Lymph drainage occurs towards the hilum via vessels which lie close to the bronchi or form a pleural network. Lymph flow is promoted by the constant movement of adjacent structures and is rendered unidirectional by numerous valves. The lymph finally drains into the venous system mainly via the right lymphatic duct and the thoracic duct, although there is also a maze of interconnecting mediastinal, paratracheal and diaphragmatic channels.

Extensive lymphoid tissue is found in the lungs. Submucosal aggregations occur as far as the respiratory bronchioles distally and true lymph nodes from the segmental bronchi proximally. A large group of nodes is clustered about each hilum and these connect with adjacent para-aortic, paratracheal and mediastinal nodes.

Chest wall

The chest wall is based on a bony and cartilaginous framework of encircling ribs, articulated posteriorly with the thoracic spine and anteriorly with the sternum. Between the ribs lie the external and internal intercostal muscles. The thoracic and abdominal contents are separated by the diaphragm.

A thin but continuous serous membrane covers the external surfaces of the lungs (the visceral pleura) and the internal surfaces of the chest wall, diaphragm and mediastinum (the parietal pleura). The pleura consists of a single layer of flat, mesothelial cells without a basement membrane. The underlying connective tissue contains abundant blood vessels and lymphatics. Unlike the parietal pleura, the visceral pleura has no sensory nerve endings and is closely adherent to its underlying structures. The pleural space is only a potential one, since the visceral and parietal pleural surfaces are normally apposed, apart from a thin film of fluid which provides lubrication and permits easy movement of the two surfaces in relation to each other.

Respiratory muscles

The main respiratory muscles are the diaphragm and intercostal muscles. The diaphragm is a large, powerful and complex musculotendinous sheet. It is a dome-shaped structure which attaches peripherally by muscular fibres to the vertebral bodies, ribs and sternum, and ends centrally in a fibrous sheet called the central tendon. In addition to an hiatus each for the oesophagus, aorta and inferior vena cava, other pleuroperitoneal foramina are sometimes present.

The excursion of the diaphragm during breathing varies from 1.5–10 cm and is responsible for about 75% of the volume of inspiration. Diaphragmatic contraction pulls the central tendon downwards, since the peripheral attachments remain relatively fixed, although the costal margin is partly raised and everted at this time. These actions elongate the thoracic cavity and expand its volume. Abnormalities of position and function of the diaphragm are common in a large number of disease states.

The intercostal muscles function primarily in inspiration, when they are responsible for about 25% of the volume inspired. Accessory muscles of respiration, such as the sternomastoids, are usually active only during deep breathing. Expiration is normally passive and produced by the elastic recoil of the lungs. However, in obstructed breathing, expiration may be assisted by part of the internal intercostal muscles and

9/*Structure of the Respiratory System*

by the abdominal muscles. The latter are, of course, also important in coughing and straining.

Innervation

The lungs are innervated via the vagus nerves and the upper six thoracic sympathetic ganglia. Autonomic fibres form a plexus surrounding the airways as far as the bronchioles. The parasympathetic efferents produce bronchial smooth muscle contraction, blood vessel dilatation and mucous gland secretion. The sympathetic efferents produce bronchial smooth muscle dilatation.

Parasympathetic afferents carry impulses from the pulmonary stretch receptors situated in the walls of the main airways, from cough and irritant receptors in the mucosa of the larger airways and from receptors (J receptors) in the alveolar interstitium. Other respiratory reflexes include pulmonary vascular responses (e.g. to embolism), possible pulmonary chemoreceptors, and protective upper airway responses such as sneezing, coughing and gagging. There are also numerous pathways from somatic and visceral receptors which chiefly give local and systemic responses in various parts of the body but which may also give respiratory responses such as gasping.

Somatic motor nerves (phrenic and intercostal) supply the muscles of respiration and somatic sensory nerves (phrenic, intercostal and spinal) innervate the chest wall, including the parietal pleura.

2   Respiratory Physiology

Introduction

The chief function of the lungs is gas exchange. This refers to the transfer of oxygen and carbon dioxide between the environment and the blood. In addition to gas exchange, the lungs are also involved in the regulation of the acid—base state and in a number of non-respiratory functions.

Gas exchange is conveniently divided into four processes, namely ventilation, gas transfer, pulmonary blood flow and blood gas transport.

Ventilation

Ventilation results from the rhythmic contraction of the inspiratory muscles which causes expansion of the thorax and thus of the lungs. This rhythmic contraction originates in the brain stem. The level of ventilation is adjusted in response to blood oxygen and carbon dioxide tensions, which in turn depend upon the relation between ventilation and the metabolic activity of the body. Ventilatory control is thus a servo or feedback mechanism.

A normal adult at rest might typically have a total ventilation of 7.5 l/min, based on a tidal volume of 500 ml and a respiratory rate of 15 breaths/min ($\dot{V}_E = V_T \times f$). Since the anatomical dead-space (volume of conducting airways) is about 140 ml (2 ml/kg), the ventilation actually reaching the alveoli is only about 5.5 l/min (360 ml x 15 breaths/min) [$\dot{V}_A = (V_T - V_D) \times f$]. If the tidal volume decreases, the proportion of ventilation that is solely dead-space ventilation also increases.

Parts of the lung which have reduced or absent blood flow also behave as dead-space, since the air going to those parts can perform little or no gas exchange. This alveolar dead-space plus the anatomical dead-space comprise the total or physiological dead-space (V_D). In normal subjects, the physiological dead-space is the same as the anatomical dead-space, since there is little or no alveolar dead-space. In disease states, the alveolar dead-space may become markedly increased.

Lung volumes

The total volume of air in the lungs is subdivided into eight different components (Fig. 2.1). The most important of these are:

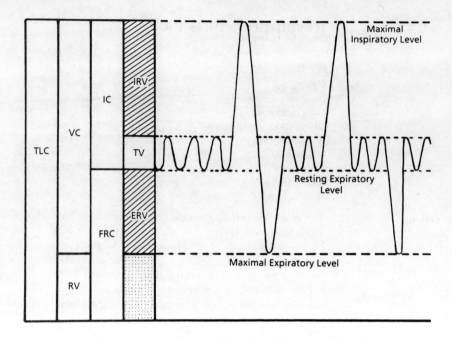

Fig. 2.1. Subdivisions of lung volumes. IC = inspiratory capacity. IRV = inspiratory reserve volume. ERV = expiratory reserve volume. See text for other components. (From Cade, 1984.)

- *tidal volume* (V_T or TV), which is the volume of air inspired or expired during breathing;
- *vital capacity* (VC), which is the volume of air expelled by maximum expiration after maximum inspiration;
- *functional residual capacity* (FRC), which is the volume of air remaining in the lungs at the end of normal expiration;
- *residual volume* (RV), which is the volume of air remaining in the lungs after maximal expiration; and
- *total lung capacity* (TLC), which is the volume of air in the lungs at maximum inspiration.

Lung mechanics

The mechanical function of the lungs describes those properties which determine the volume and distribution of ventilation following a given inspiratory stimulus. The mechanical properties of the lungs can be considered in two situations, namely with static forces acting at fixed lung volumes and with dynamic forces acting during airflow. The former are elastic forces and the latter include both elastic and resistive forces.

The *elastic* properties of the lungs, commonly referred to as compliance, describe the change in lung volume for a given change in distending pressure. Although compliance varies in a non-linear fashion with changing lung volume, a single value called specific compliance can be calculated by relating the compliance to the size of the FRC. The most comprehensive way of viewing compliance is to examine the pressure–volume curve of inflation and deflation over the entire range of lung volume (Fig. 2.2). The shape of this pressure–volume curve is an overall result of lung distensibility.

The distensibility of the lungs derives not only from the elastic tissues themselves, but also particularly from the surface tension of the liquid lining of the alveoli. While the small size of the alveoli minimizes the distance that gases have to diffuse and maximizes the area of the alveolar surface, the pressure generated by surface tension becomes greater as the radius of the alveoli becomes smaller (Laplace's law). Fortunately, the surface tension of the air–liquid interface which lines the alveoli is reduced many times compared with that of an air–water interface by the presence of surfactant. Surface tension is different in an inflating lung compared with a deflating lung and this largely explains the different pressure-volume curves for inflation and deflation (hysteresis) (Fig. 2.2).

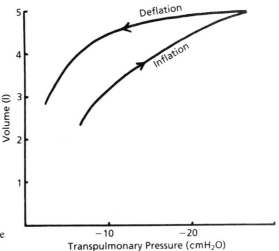

Fig. 2.2. Transpulmonary pressure/lung volume relationships over the range of breathing.

Resistive forces are determined by the pressure gradient along the airways and the rate of airflow. The pressure gradient in turn depends on the length and especially the calibre of the airways and the viscosity of the gas involved. Airflow at many sites in the respiratory tract is turbulent rather than laminar, so that an increase in airflow entails a disproportionate increase in pressure gradient and therefore resistive work. It is thus not possible to give a single value for airway resistance that covers all rates and volumes of breathing. For practical purposes, however, airway resistance is calculated from measurements made during quiet, tidal breathing. Most of the total airway resistance arises from the larger airways. The resistance of the small airways and of other lung tissues is very small.

Expiration is normally produced by the recoil of the stretched elastic tissues of the lungs. During forced expiration, the intrathoracic or intrapleural pressure becomes positive because of muscular effort. There comes a point when increasing muscular effort tends to compress the airway and not increase the rate of airflow. The expiratory flow-rate during forced expiration thus becomes 'effort-independent' and is determined by the elastic recoil pressure and the resistance of the small airways. Any reduction in calibre of these airways predisposes to premature closure and air trapping.

Distribution of ventilation

The distribution of ventilation within the lungs may become uneven for two reasons. Firstly, there are regional differences in distending pressure in both health and disease. Thus there is a gradient of intrapleural pressure down the lung, so that the pressure is about 7.5 cm of water less at the top of the lung than at the bottom. The transpulmonary pressure and the recoil pressure therefore increase from the bottom to the top of the lung. As a result, the top of the lung operates on a flatter part of the pressure–volume curve than the bottom of the lung and receives less ventilation during normal breathing.

Secondly, there are local differences in mechanical factors which occur in many disease states. The local compliance determines the volume of ventilation received by a lung unit. Its airway resistance determines the rate of ventilation. The product of compliance and resistance, sometimes referred to as the *time constant*, determines the amount of ventilation in a given time. Unequal time constants of different lung units give rise to uneven distribution of ventilation. This unevenness becomes more marked with increasing respiratory rate (Fig. 2.3).

Respiratory work

The mechanical work of breathing is calculated from measurements of transpulmonary pressure and ventilation. In normal subjects, the total mechanical work of breathing is about 0.6 kp m/min (0.1 W), of which at least two-thirds is expended on the lungs and the remainder on the chest wall. In patients with lung disease, the mechanical work of breathing may be increased up to 10-fold or more. The metabolic cost of breathing can be estimated from the oxygen consumption of the respiratory muscles. This is normally 1–3% of the total oxygen consumption, or about 4 ml O_2/min. Even during strenuous exercise, the oxygen consumption of the respiratory muscles in normal subjects still represents only a small proportion of the total oxygen uptake. However, in patients with heart or lung disease, the oxygen consumption of the respiratory muscles during exercise may reach such high levels as to restrict quite severely the amount of oxygen available to the rest of the body.

Gas transfer

The exchange of oxygen and carbon dioxide between the air in the alveoli and the blood in the pulmonary capillaries depends on the appropriate distribution of ventilation and

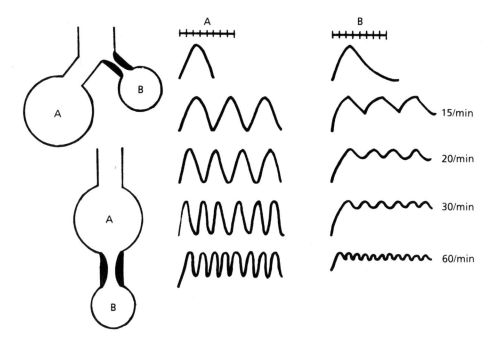

Fig. 2.3. The influence of increasing respiratory frequency on the non-uniformity of ventilation between two compartments with unequal time constants (A and B, in parallel or in series). The amplitude of the tracings reflects the amount of ventilation.

blood flow, the diffusion of gases through the alveolar air and the various membranes and liquid layers, and chemical reactions within the red cells.

Of greater functional importance than either the distribution of ventilation or the distribution of blood flow is the distribution of ventilation relative to blood flow. Areas which have much greater ventilation than blood flow behave as dead-space and areas with much greater blood flow than ventilation behave as right-to-left shunt. This is represented in Fig. 2.4 in which the homogeneous situation of uniform ventilation and blood flow is shown as a single gas exchanging unit (a). Excessive ventilation in relation to blood flow and excessive blood flow in relation to ventilation (b) are the two situations of ventilation/blood flow inhomogeneity. They may be modelled conceptually as increased (alveolar) dead-space and right-to-left shunt, respectively (c). Unless the proportion of ventilation to blood flow in all alveoli is both uniform and appropriate to the mixed venous and inspired gas compositions, the arterial blood gas composition cannot be normal. In other words, ventilation/blood flow inequality must result in abnormal arterial blood gas values.

Although over-ventilated alveoli can excrete more carbon dioxide and thus tend to compensate for the carbon dioxide retention in under-ventilated alveoli, they cannot completely

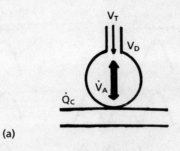

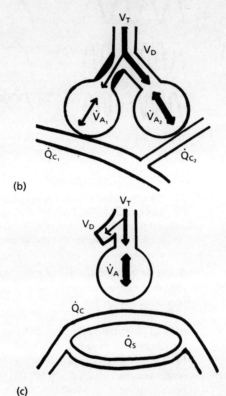

Fig. 2.4. Models of alveolar ventilation/pulmonary blood flow distribution.
(a) Homogeneity.
(b) Inhomogeneity.
(c) Inhomogeneity represented as a three compartment model with dead-space (V_D) and right-to-left shunt ($\dot{Q}_s$).

compensate for inequality of oxygen uptake. This is because over-ventilation gives rise to only a small increase in the quantity of oxygen taken up due to the shape of the oxygen dissociation curve. The only way in which oxygenation may be corrected in the presence of ventilation/blood flow inequality is for total ventilation to increase. This increases ventilation in the relatively under-ventilated alveoli and so increases their ventilation/blood flow ratios. However, since increased total ventilation must also increase ventilation in those alveoli already over-ventilated, there must be a reduction in the arterial carbon dioxide tension. Thus, the final result of hyper-ventilation in the face of ventilation/blood flow inequality is improvement in and possible normalization of the arterial oxygen tension, but at the expense of a lowered arterial carbon dioxide tension; there remains a widened alveolar-arterial oxygen tension gradient.

Although ventilation moves the gases in bulk up and down the airways, their movement in the depths of the lung is by molecular diffusion. Oxygen and carbon dioxide diffuse at almost equal rates in the gas phase but, because of its greater solubility, carbon dioxide diffuses through the aqueous layers and membranes more readily than oxygen. However, even for oxygen, there is virtually no diffusion barrier between the alveolar air and the red cell, even during stresses such as exercise or disease. The absence of an alveolar to end-capillary gradient for oxygen should be distinguished from the alveolar-arterial oxygen tension difference, which is primarily due to ventilation/blood flow inequality.

The final step in gas transfer involves a number of chemical reactions within the red cell. The volume of oxygen taken up is determined by the rate of combination of oxygen with haemoglobin and the volume of haemoglobin present. Carbon dioxide is formed by the dehydration of carbonic acid, a reaction which is catalyzed by carbonic anhydrase.

Pulmonary blood flow

The distribution of blood flow within the lung is determined chiefly by gravity. Thus blood flow is considerably greater at the base than at the apex of the lung. However, the rate of increasing blood flow down the lung is not linear but depends on the interrelations between pulmonary arterial, pulmonary venous and alveolar pressures (Fig. 2.5).

● In *zone one* at the top of the lung, arterial pressure is less

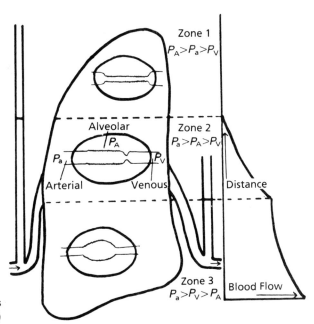

Fig. 2.5. The influence on local blood flow within the lung of the relationships between local alveolar, arterial and venous pressures (redrawn from West, 1985b.)

than alveolar pressure and there is no blood flow. Zone one is small in normal subjects, even at rest.

• In *zone two* in the middle of the lung, arterial pressure is greater than alveolar pressure, which in turn is greater than venous pressure. In this situation, the driving pressure is the arterial-alveolar difference.

• In *zone three* at the base of the lung, the venous pressure is now greater than the alveolar pressure and the driving pressure is the arterial-venous difference.

Although the factors determining the distribution of blood flow in the lung have been elucidated by studying the erect subject, the same principles apply in any other position, except that the effect of gravity operates over a smaller vertical gradient.

The matching of the distribution of blood flow to the distribution of ventilation is maintained by a number of homeostatic mechanisms. Thus, if local ventilation is impaired, compensatory reduction in blood flow tends to occur. This is mediated via local hypoxic vasoconstriction. This mechanism explains the fall in arterial oxygen tension sometimes seen following the administration of bronchodilators. This is because these agents are also vasodilators and vasodilatation generally occurs before bronchodilatation, so that temporary worsening of ventilation/blood flow matching follows. A second mechanism may operate in areas of severe obstruction where local hyperinflation may cause stretching, flattening and mechanical obstruction of the capillaries in the alveolar walls, so that for anatomical reasons blood flow may be reduced in areas of poor local ventilation.

Conversely, if local blood flow is impaired, mechanisms also exist which tend to reduce local ventilation. For example, vascular obstruction results not only in alveolar hypocapnia which can produce bronchoconstriction, but also in impaired production of surfactant which can lead to alveolar collapse. Moreover, vascular obstruction due to pulmonary embolism may be associated with the release, for example from platelets, of bronchoactive and vasoactive substances, such as histamine, serotonin, prostaglandins and leucotrienes.

The lung thus has a remarkable series of local regulatory mechanisms, which are capable of maintaining the matching of ventilation and blood flow, even in the presence of considerable maldistribution of air or blood. These mechanisms, however, are not perfect enough to compensate completely for abnormal local ventilation or blood flow, so that some or even considerable ventilation/blood flow inequality always remains in these situations.

Blood gas transport

The relation between the partial pressure of oxygen and the volume of oxygen carried in the blood is given by the dissociation curve (Fig. 2.6). Clinically, the shape of the curve is important in several ways. Firstly, even considerable reduction in oxygen tension below the normal arterial range (80–

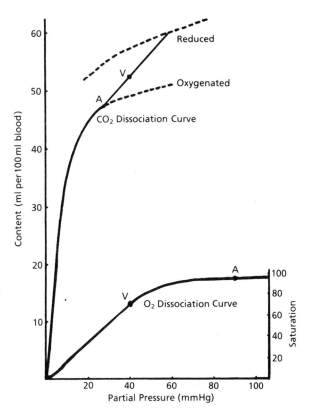

Fig. 2.6.Oxygen and carbon dioxide dissociation curves of blood. V and A represent approximate values for normal mixed venous and arterial blood respectively in resting man. The influence of oxygenation of blood on its carbon dioxide carrying ability is shown and explains why V and A are not on a single carbon dioxide dissociation curve. The effect of carbon dioxide addition or removal on oxygen transport is much less and is not shown. Note that the oxygen content level (unlike the oxygen saturation) at any gas tension depends on the haemoglobin concentration, the values shown being for a normal haemoglobin concentration. (Redrawn from Cade, 1984.)

100 mmHg) does not significantly reduce the oxygenation of arterial blood. Thus, the saturation does not fall below 90% until the tension has fallen below 60 mmHg. Secondly, the change in shape below 60 mmHg means that further reductions in tension are associated with large falls in saturation. This permits ready unloading of oxygen in the tissues.

The shape of the oxygen dissociation curve is affected by a number of physiological variables. Increased carbon dioxide tension, hydrogen ion concentration, temperature, and the red cell concentrations of certain organic phosphates, notably 2,3-diphosphoglycerate (2,3-DPG), all shift the curve to the right, thereby facilitating the unloading of oxygen in the tissues. The opposite changes shift the curve to the left, thereby hindering the unloading of oxygen in the tissues. In chronic hypoxia, the concentration of 2,3-DPG is increased, whereas in carbon monoxide poisoning, transfusion of stored blood, metabolic acidosis, and some rare red cell enzyme defects, its concentration is decreased. The position of the oxygen dissociation curve is expressed as the P_{50}, namely the oxygen tension at 50% saturation. The normal P_{50} is about 27 mmHg.

Carbon dioxide is carried in the blood in simple solution, as bicarbonate and combined with protein, chiefly haemoglobin in the form of carbamino compounds. As the blood passes along the tissue capillaries, dissolved carbon dioxide diffuses through the plasma and into the red cells, where carbonic anhydrase accelerates the formation of carbonic acid. The carbonic acid dissociates into hydrogen and bicarbonate ions. The hydrogen ions are buffered by haemoglobin and the bicarbonate ions diffuse out into the plasma and are replaced by chloride ions which enter the cell to restore equilibrium. In the pulmonary capillaries, these processes are reversed. The relation between the partial pressure of carbon dioxide and the volume of carbon dioxide carried in the blood is given by its dissociation curve (Fig. 2.6). Unlike the oxygen dissociation curve, that for carbon dioxide does not reach a plateau. Thus, over-ventilation of parts of the lung can remove carbon dioxide to help compensate for under-ventilation of other parts of the lung. Because of the shape of the oxygen dissociation curve, little such compensation for local variations in ventilation can occur for oxygen, as previously discussed.

The body contains 'stores' of about one litre of oxygen and 17 litres of carbon dioxide, excluding the gases in the lungs. Most of the oxygen is in the blood, whereas the bulk of the carbon dioxide is in the tissue fluids as bicarbonate. These differences in storage capacity and distribution are of considerable clinical importance. Changes in the volume of ventilation or the composition of the inspired air alter the oxygen stores within two minutes, whereas the carbon dioxide stores take more than 15 min to reach their new level.

The clinical significance of these differences is illustrated by the patient who has under-ventilated while breathing oxygen. If he is now given air to breathe instead of oxygen, the oxygen tension in the blood and tissues falls rapidly. Increasing the ventilation back to normal, however, cannot completely counteract this fall, because the high partial pressure of carbon dioxide which now exists in the mixed venous blood maintains the alveolar carbon dioxide tension high for several minutes, thus diluting the oxygen in the alveolar air. The maintenance of a normal alveolar oxygen concentration during this time will require considerable over-ventilation, which may be beyond the ventilatory capacity of such a patient. The resultant hypoxaemia can be considerable and may be worse than before oxygen was given in the first place.

Control of breathing

The rhythm of breathing is generated in the pons and medulla in a group of neurones customarily referred to as the 'respiratory centre'. In man, the rhythmicity probably depends on chemical and other neural inputs and is not intrinsic. The volume of breathing is determined chiefly by chemical stimuli in the blood and the pattern of breathing by mechanical stimuli relayed in the vagus nerve from the lung. The most important chemical stimulus is the arterial carbon dioxide tension as sensed by the medullary chemoreceptors. Ventilation is normally adjusted to keep the arterial carbon dioxide at about 40 mmHg. Chemoreceptors in the aortic and carotid bodies respond to hypoxaemia so as to stimulate ventilation but only when the arterial oxygen tension falls below about 60 mmHg.

The medullary or central chemoreceptors can have their sensitivity temporarily or chronically reset in either direction. Firstly, when ventilation is chronically increased, for example by the hypoxia of altitude or by a mechanical ventilator, the medullary chemoreceptors become adjusted down to the lower carbon dioxide tension and will then resist any tendency for it to rise. Thus, patients who are chronically over-ventilated by a ventilator can become distressed if ventilation is acutely reduced, even though the arterial oxygen tension remains normal and the carbon dioxide tension below normal. Secondly, faced with a chronically high carbon dioxide tension, as occurs in some cases of chronic lung disease, the medullary chemoreceptors can be adjusted up to the higher carbon dioxide tension and can lose their sensitivity to its change. The ventilation may then be maintained largely by hypoxic drive of the peripheral chemoreceptors. Administration of oxygen to such patients will abolish this drive with the result that ventilation can become severely reduced and the carbon dioxide tension can rise to narcotic levels without the normal stimulation of a central chemoreceptor drive to breathe.

Although the precise mechanisms are unknown, the pattern of breathing is adjusted to minimize the work required. Airway calibre is also subject to a fine adjustment, whereby the autonomic nervous system by its control of bronchial smooth muscle tone maintains an optimal balance between the resistance and the dead-space of the airways. The final result of these mechanisms is that for any given combination of compliance, resistance and dead-space, there is an optimal combination of rate and depth of breathing for each level of alveolar ventilation. The frequency of breathing of normal subjects is close to this optimum and the abnormal ventilatory patterns seen in many disease states, for example in conditions of reduced compliance, also approximate an optimum.

Exercise

The chief changes in respiratory function during exercise are increases in ventilation and blood flow (cardiac output). The typical magnitude of changes in these and other important variables during heavy exercise (e.g. about 1800 kp m/min or 300 W) in a healthy subject are shown in Table 2.1. Ventilation (minute volume) increases over 10-fold, pulmonary blood flow 6-fold, and oxygen uptake and carbon dioxide output 16-fold. The arterial oxygen tension may fall slightly and the carbon dioxide tension usually falls. There is a metabolic acidosis due to an increase in blood lactate. The rate of change of these variables is not linearly related to the intensity of the physical work as judged by the carbon dioxide output. Thus, ventilation increases in proportion during light and moderate exercise but increases disproportionately during severe exercise, chiefly because of the development of acidosis.

A corollary of this excessive ventilation is that the arterial carbon dioxide tension is lower during severe exercise than during moderate exercise.

Table 2.1. Typical changes after heavy exercise

Variable	Rest	Exercise
$\dot{V}_E$ (l/min)	8	>100
C.O. (l/min)	5	30
$\dot{V}o_2$ (l/min)	0.25	4
$\dot{V}co_2$ (l/min)	0.25	4
P_ao_2		slight fall
P_aco_2		fall
pH	7.40	7.30
Blood lactate (mmol/l)	<1	>10

In all exercise lasting more than a minute or so, the rate of work is limited by the subject's capacity to exchange and transport oxygen and carbon dioxide. Limitations can occur in the capacity of any of the links in the chain of respiratory and circulatory functions connecting the tissues with the air:

1 Inability to increase ventilation in proportion to carbon dioxide output and oxygen uptake causes the alveolar and arterial carbon dioxide tension to rise and the alveolar and arterial oxygen tension to fall. Usually dyspnoea caused by the ventilatory stimulus of a rising carbon dioxide tension causes the subject to stop before significant hypoxaemia develops, provided the initial arterial oxygen tension is not already reduced.

2 Inability to increase the capacity of the lungs to transfer oxygen in proportion to an increase in oxygen uptake causes an increased alveolar-arterial oxygen tension difference. The fall in arterial oxygen tension causes a further increase in ventilation and cardiac output.

3 Inability to increase cardiac output in proportion to carbon dioxide output or oxygen uptake causes a widened veno-arterial difference for carbon dioxide and oxygen and a fall in tissue oxygen tension. This may cause an increase in anaerobic metabolism.

4 The effect of anaemia is similar with respect to oxygen to a reduction in cardiac output, in that the supply of oxygen to the tissues is reduced. The important difference, however, is that in anaemia the cardiac output is usually increased.

5 Inability of the muscles and their vascular bed to increase their capacity to transfer oxygen in proportion to an increased oxygen usage, or an enzymatic limitation in the ability of the muscle cells to take up oxygen, causes an increased difference in oxygen tension between the blood and the tissues and may cause an increase in anaerobic metabolism. The difference between this form of limitation and a reduction in cardiac output is that the arteriovenous oxygen difference is not increased in this situation.

If the processes above are unable to increase the supply of oxygen to the exercising muscles in proportion to their energy consumption, excessive anaerobic metabolism occurs, causing the addition of lactic acid to the tissue fluid. In addition, excessive demands on local muscle groups may cause local symptoms. Symptoms of local significance, such as angina pectoris, intermittent claudication or wheeze, may be responsible for limitation of exercise tolerance. However, in unfitness and in most disease states, such as heart disease, lung disease and anaemia, the limit is signalled by breathlessness. This is because whatever site is involved by disease in the chain of respiratory and circulatory processes, there is commonly an increased drive to breathe from an increased carbon dioxide load and from a variety of other stimuli.

Non-respiratory functions   Although the chief function of the lungs is gas exchange (or 'external respiration'), they are also involved in a number of other functions. Lung defences involved in conditioning of the inhaled air, heat and water exchange during expiration, and inhaled particle clearance, have been described in the previous chapter on the structure of the respiratory system. The lungs also act as a filter of particular matter from the systemic venous system, thus protecting other organs, such as the brain, from the hazards of embolization. Only a very small proportion of particles larger than red blood cells pass through the pulmonary capillary bed. It is likely that filtration is a continuously operative function even in health and is not confined to disease states. The lung itself tolerates embolism better than other organs because of its dual blood supply and its very efficient disposal mechanisms.

The lungs also have important roles in metabolism (especially of lipids), in activation and deactivation of many biologically active substances (such as serotonin, histamine, catecholamines, angiotensin, polypeptide hormones, prostaglandins, leucotrienes), in trapping and release of formed elements, and as a potential reservoir of blood to maintain left ventricular filling on a short-term basis. The role of the lungs in the metabolism of angiotensin is of particular importance, since the pulmonary endothelial cells are the main site in the body of converting enzyme. This converts the relatively inactive decapeptide, angiotensin I (derived from the action of renin on angiotensinogen), into the highly potent octapeptide, angiotensin II, within a single pass through the pulmonary circulation.

Symbols   Like other specialties, respiratory physiology has become associated with the use of shorthand symbols which, once understood, make the description of relationships much easier. The list in Table 2.2, although not exhaustive, should be sufficient to explain the logic and to be of practical help. Abbreviations are not listed as they are explained when first encountered in the text and are included in the index.

Table 2.2. Common symbols used in respiratory physiology

Quantities (primary symbols)

C	content of gas in a liquid
D	diffusing capacity (diffusing capability, diffusion constant, diffusivity)
F	fractional concentration of a gas
P	pressure (partial pressure of a subscripted gas or absolute pressure of a liquid as vertical height of liquid column)
Pa	partial pressure of a gas or absolute pressure of liquid in Pascals
Q	blood volume
S	saturation of haemoglobin with a specified gas
V	gas volume

Flow rates

$\dot{Q}$	blood flow per unit time
$\dot{V}$	ventilation (gas flow) per unit time; gas produced or consumed per unit time

Descriptive subscripts

A	alveolar gas
E	expired gas
$\overline{E}$	mixed expired gas
I	inspired gas
a	arterial blood
c	capillary blood
$\bar{c}$	mean capillary blood
v	venous blood
$\bar{v}$	mixed venous blood
s	shunt
t	total
D	dead-space
T	tidal

Examples

$\dot{V}_A/\dot{Q}_c$	ratio of alveolar ventilation to pulmonary capillary blood flow
$C_{\bar{v}}O_2$	oxygen content of mixed venous blood
F_IO_2	fractional concention of inspired oxygen
$\dot{Q}_s/\dot{Q}_t$	shunt blood flow in relation to total blood flow
V_D/V_T	ratio of dead-space volume to tidal volume

Respiratory Symptoms and Signs

Introduction

The history and the physical examination are as integral a part of respiratory assessment as they are for any other branch of clinical medicine. History taking is important in a number of ways. Firstly, symptoms are usually the reason for the patient's presentation and need to be clarified in their own right. Secondly, the findings on initial interview are usually chiefly responsible for the direction of subsequent investigations. Thirdly, a careful history may sometimes be the prime route to much or all of the final diagnosis. Fourthly, only the history is able to quantify satisfactorily many respiratory disabilities and thus guide both therapy and prognosis.

In obtaining the history, questions should always be asked concerning childhood ailments, family history, current and past smoking habits, current and previous occupations, environmental exposure, pets (especially birds), drugs, leisure activities and travel. A comprehensive general medical history should always be taken, both because some systemic diseases have respiratory components and because many respiratory diseases have systemic consequences. The cardinal respiratory symptoms relate to cough, breathlessness and chest pain.

Cough

Cough is a non-specific symptom but should always be regarded as abnormal. During a cough, the glottis is initially closed until the expiratory muscles have built up appropriate positive pressure. The glottis is then opened and the resulting explosive force greatly increases the linear velocity of airflow. The linear velocity may reach Mach 1 (nearly 1000 km/hr) in the trachea and is well designed to expel material from the lumen or shear it off the walls of the airways.

Cough and irritant receptors are present in the major airways, as previously discussed. The chief function of coughing is thus to clear material from the central part of the tracheobronchial tree. This material may be either excessive secretions or foreign matter. Secretions are normally dealt with by the mucociliary transport system discussed previously and do not produce coughing unless they are quite excessive. Foreign material, either particulate, liquid or gaseous, also stimulates coughing as a defensive mechanism.

The cough receptors can also be stimulated by irritant

mechanisms which have nothing to do with airway defence. Thus, inflammation or tumour may give rise to unproductive coughing which is often prolonged and distressing. Severe bouts of coughing, particularly if dry and irritating, may give rise to exhaustion, vomiting, syncope or even rib fractures. A productive cough implies the presence of sputum or blood (haemoptysis).

Sputum

Sputum is the production of tracheobronchial secretions which are excessive and are expelled by coughing. Genuine sputum, coughed from the chest, must be distinguished from saliva and nasal and pharyngeal secretions which may be spat. The quantity and nature of sputum is of considerable diagnostic importance. Large amounts of sputum are seen in chronic bronchitis and bronchiectasis, and also in non-inflammatory conditions such as alveolar cell carcinoma. Yellow or green sputum is typically associated with respiratory infection, foul-smelling sputum with lung abscess often due to anaerobes, pink frothy sputum with acute pulmonary oedema, rusty sputum with serious pneumonia, and tenacious sputum especially if mucoid with asthma.

Haemoptysis

Haemoptysis, or the expectoration of blood, should always be regarded as potentially serious. Haemoptysis may range from minor blood streaking of the sputum to the expectoration of large amounts of frank blood. Most haemoptysis is minor, but even relatively small amounts of blood can be quite startling when mixed with expectorated sputum. The source of expectorated blood is not always clear from the history. Blood from the mouth, nose or throat, or the upper gastrointestinal tract, may well into the throat and then be coughed up. Patients, and even clinicians, may also have difficulty sometimes in distinguishing between haemoptysis and haematemesis. Some degree of haemoptysis is common with many acute respiratory infections, though most causes of haemoptysis are serious chronic diseases, such as carcinoma, tuberculosis, bronchiectasis and mitral stenosis. The chief causes of haemoptysis are listed in Chapter 21 (Table 21.3).

Dyspnoea

Shortness of breath (dyspnoea, breathlessness) can be one of the most distressing of clinical symptoms. Dyspnoea describes the sensation of excessive awareness of breathing or actual discomfort in its act. Many non-respiratory as well as respiratory mechanisms can lead to dyspnoea and similarly, many of the responses to dyspnoea are systemic or non-respiratory.

The exact mechanism or mechanisms of dyspnoea are not completely understood and there are probably several. The most important may be the sensation of an imbalance or inappropriateness between the volume or flow of ventilation demanded and the forces required to meet that demand. This is the main sensation giving rise to dyspnoea in lung or heart disease and is associated with changes in the mechanical state of the lungs or chest wall. An increased amount or rate of ventilation (hyperpnoea or tachypnoea), for example in anaemia or metabolic acidosis, may sometimes be uncomfortable. Mostly, however, such sensations are of importance chiefly in their ability to aggravate or magnify the sensation of inappropriateness produced by another condition. In addition, discomfort may also arise from irritation or spasm in the major central airways or perhaps from receptors in pulmonary arteries. These mechanisms may contribute to the dyspnoea associated with asthma and pulmonary embolism, respectively. Ventilation is elegantly balanced to maintain oxygen and carbon dioxide exchange under conditions of greatly varying demand. However, chemical disturbances in the blood acting through the chemoreceptors, or mechanical changes in the lungs acting through the vagi, are important only as sources of inspiratory drive and not of sensation. The sensations responsible for the symptom of dyspnoea are associated rather with the motor response to the respiratory drive.

Dyspnoea is usually most marked on exertion. Sometimes it may be associated with wheeze, as in exercise-induced asthma. Sometimes it occurs predominantly at rest, particularly in the recumbent position when it is referred to as orthopnoea. Orthopnoea is due to an increase in pulmonary blood volume causing a reduction in compliance, though other factors such as disturbed ventilation/blood flow ratios, mechanical disadvantage of respiratory muscles, particularly the diaphragm, and reflex mechanisms may also be important. The elucidation of dyspnoea requires a careful history of its course and associated circumstances, as well as appropriate subsequent investigations. The chief causes of dyspnoea are listed in Chapter 21 (Table 21.1).

Chest pain

Chest pain is a common respiratory symptom and may be of various types. The commonest types are pleuritic, chest wall, and cardiac. Many major structures within the chest are insensitive to pain. Thus, pain stimuli do not arise from the lung itself or the visceral pleura, though they do arise from the parietal pleura, major airways, chest wall, diaphragm and mediastinum.

● *Pleuritic pain*, originating from the parietal pleura, may be quite severe. It is usually relatively localized and characteristically is exacerbated by and limits full inspiration. It is also aggravated by coughing and movement. It may be especially associated with pulmonary infections, carcinoma or embolism.

● *Chest wall pain* includes muscular pain, intercostal neuritis (for example, from herpes zoster) or costochondritis. Less commonly, chest wall pain may be due to previously unrecognized rib fractures or other trauma, disorders of the thoracic spine, or rheumatic pains involving the muscles, fascia and joints of the chest wall.

● Important causes of pain in the chest which may sometimes mimic respiratory disease include pain of cardiac or pericardial origin, oesophageal pain or occasionally pain associated with dissecting thoracic aneurysm. Conversely, central chest discomfort, especially on inspiration, occurs in tracheobronchitis and may occasionally be mistaken for cardiac or oesophageal pain.

Wheeze and stridor

Noisy breathing may be a prominent respiratory complaint but is more often an associated symptom uncovered during history taking or on clinical examination.
• *Wheeze* is caused by narrowing of the major intrathoracic airways and this gives rise to limitation of airflow, particularly during expiration. Expiration is thus noisy and squeaky, prolonged and sometimes distressing. Although most conditions giving rise to wheeze are diffuse, wheeze may sometimes be due to local obstruction, such as by tumour or foreign body. The time-course of wheeze, its other associations and its potential reversibility are important aspects to be elucidated in the history. The chief causes of wheeze are listed in Chapter 21 (Table 21.2).
• *Stridor* is caused by narrowing of the major extrathoracic airways, especially the larynx, and gives rise to limitation of airflow, particularly during inspiration. Acute infections (especially in children) and recent trauma are major causes. Other less common causes include acute allergic reactions, malignancy and extrinsic compression.

Physical examination

The physical examination of the chest is not time-consuming but should be done according to a protocol so that nothing is missed. A complete general examination should also be performed for the same reasons that a complete general history should always be taken. While positive physical findings are important, their absence does not exclude significant respiratory disease. A chest X-ray is therefore an essential extension of the initial examination. The signs elicited on physical examination are rarely specific or diagnostic but are major clues in clarifying the patient's problem and in both suggesting appropriate further investigations and understanding their results. The examination should allow decisions concerning the normality or otherwise of the lungs and the likely nature and severity of any pathological process. The techniques of lung examination are best taught by bedside instruction and reinforced by rigorous practice. The classical progression through inspection, palpation, percussion and auscultation has much to offer in chest examination.
• *Inspection* may reveal much about the patient even before the specific examination of the chest begins. The presence, for example, of breathlessness, wheeze, cough, sighing, plethora or cyanosis may have been noted during interview. Inspection of the chest should include shape and symmetry of the thoracic cage, the amount and symmetry of respiratory excursions, the presence of rib retraction, surgical or other scars, the shape and mobility of the thoracic spine and, in women, the breasts.

• *Palpation* of the lower chest from behind helps clarify the extent and symmetry of chest expansion. The position of the trachea should be felt in the suprasternal notch, where it is normally central, and combined with detection of the position of the apex beat, it provides information about mediastinal displacement. Cervical or axillary lymphadenopathy should be sought. Vocal fremitus is the transmission of voice sounds through the chest wall to the clinician's hand, most sensitively detected with the ulnar border. Vocal fremitus has the same significance as vocal resonance heard with the stethoscope, i.e. an increase suggests underlying consolidation and a decrease suggests pleural effusion.

• *Percussion* is a technique which is ideally suited for examining a gas-filled structure such as the chest and which has been most highly developed particularly for this examination. Percussion results in a complex set of signals giving the examiner both the auditory information of pitch and the tactile information of vibration or resistance, and reflects the ratio of air to solid structures under the area being percussed. The lung fields should be percussed from top to bottom, on both sides, and front and back. Cardiac percussion is not generally rewarding, apart from helping to localize the apex. Percussion gives important information on the size and symmetry of the various lung fields. Detection of the changes in the level of dullness at the bases posteriorly during breathing provides some information about diaphragmatic movement. Abnormal percussion has significance complementary to that of vocal fremitus and vocal resonance.

• *Auscultation* should be performed with the patient breathing through the mouth at a slightly increased rate and volume. The clinician listens with the diaphragm of the stethoscope over all the lung fields, starting at the top and comparing each side with the other, while moving down the lung and from the front to the back. Attention is paid to audibility and character of breath sounds, to any adventitious sounds and to voice sounds.

(a) *Breath sounds* originate in the larynx and are conducted throughout the tracheobronchial tree as far as the alveoli, thus giving information about the airways and lung tissue they traverse from their site of origin to the listener's stethoscope (Fig. 3.1).

Breath sounds heard over the larynx, trachea and large airways (centrally over the sternum and interscapular region) are characterized by a well heard inspiratory phase, a short pause (period of no airflow) and a well heard expiratory phase of the same duration as the inspiratory phase. This breath sound is abnormal if heard at more peripheral sites and is then termed *bronchial breathing*. Bronchial breathing is usually localized and signifies an area of underlying solid lung tissue (consolidation) which facilitates transmission of the sounds from the central airways.

The normal breath sound heard over the lung periphery is a

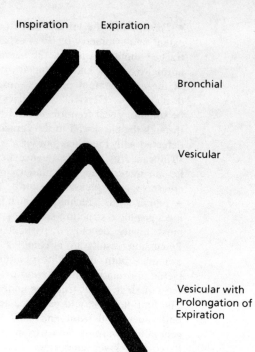

Inspiration   Expiration

Bronchial

Vesicular

Vesicular with
Prolongation of
Expiration

Breath Sounds

Fig. 3.1. Diagramatic representation of the intensity and duration of inspiratory and expiratory breath sounds. Note the gap between the end of inspiration and the beginning of expiration in bronchial breathing.

modification of the central breath sound. The pause between the inspiratory and expiratory phase is lost and the expiratory phase is shorter and softer than the inspiratory phase. This is termed *vesicular breathing*. A variant of vesicular breathing occurs when there is associated airflow obstruction so that the expiratory phase is prolonged. This breath sound is commonly mistaken for bronchial breathing.

Breath sounds, in addition to being vesicular or bronchial, may be diminished or absent, for example, if the underlying lung becomes poorly conducting because of bronchial obstruction or if there is an interposed pleural effusion or pneumothorax.

(b) *Adventitious sounds* (accompaniments) encompass the constellation of abnormal squeaking, rustling and bubbling noises which may accompany breath sounds in many respiratory disorders (Fig. 3.2). Recently, attempts have been made to provide a uniform terminology for adventitious sounds to avoid much previous confusion. *Rhonchus* (or wheeze) is suggested for continuous sounds, usually more prominent during expiration, and *crackles* for discontinuous sounds, usually more prominent during inspiration. Subclassifications with respect to pitch and coarseness are not generally helpful. Thus, the current trend is not to use terms such as crepitations, crepitant rales or discontinuous rhonchi. Technically, wheeze is an example of noisy breathing heard without a stethoscope but as it is always associated with rhonchi on auscultation, it

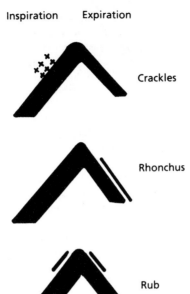

Inspiration   Expiration

Crackles

Rhonchus

Rub

Accompaniments

Fig. 3.2. Timing of accompaniments. The diagram shows the characteristic situation but accompaniments may be heard throughout both inspiration and expiration in more severely abnormal situations.

seems reasonable to use the terms wheeze and rhonchi interchangeably.

Other adventitious sounds include pleural rub, pericardial rub, pleuropericardial rub and mediastinal crunch. Pleural rub, which is particularly important in respiratory medicine, is a loud, squeaking or scratching, localized sound indicative of underlying pleural inflammation.

The mechanism of pulmonary sounds and their functional basis has been much argued but recent thinking would suggest that breath sounds transmitted through the chest wall are sounds modified as passing through a low-pass filter with a cut-off frequency greater than 200 Hz. Consolidation of lung tissue bypasses the filter. Wheezing is not due to an organ pipe effect but to the reed-like action of airways which are narrowed almost to closure and whose walls oscillate during phases of airflow, the pitch of such a wheeze being determined by the size and length of airway involved. Early inspiratory crackles are thought to be caused by the passage of a bolus of gas through an intermittently occluded airway at low lung volumes, and late inspiratory crackles are attributed to the explosive sound of previously closed peripheral airways springing open during inspiration. If adventitious sounds are heard, the patient should take a couple of deep breaths and cough. If the sounds decrease or disappear with this manoeuvre, they were due to airway secretions.

31/*Respiratory Symptoms and Signs*

(c) *Voice sounds* are the third pulmonary sounds examined during auscultation and give rise to the information called vocal resonance. The patient is asked to count or say '99' aloud and then in a whisper. The significance of vocal resonance is similar to that previously described for vocal fremitus, except that vocal resonance is probably the more sensitive technique.

Finally, auscultation of the chest for respiratory assessment is not complete without listening to the heart. The details of this examination are beyond the scope of this book but it should be emphasized that abnormalities apparent on auscultation of the left heart may be causally involved in cases of pulmonary oedema and of the right heart may be a consequence of severe respiratory disease.

Extrathoracic signs

Extrathoracic signs of respiratory disease are frequent and may provide important information not obtainable from examination of the chest alone. The hands are examined for evidence of clubbing, nicotine stains, peripheral cyanosis and osteoarthropathy; the radial pulse is checked for rate and rhythm, and the blood pressure is measured. The head and neck are then examined for plethora, central cyanosis, raised jugular venous pressure, lymphadenopathy, goitre and the position of the trachea. These areas are most conveniently examined before the chest. Afterwards, the abdomen is examined for hepatosplenomegaly, other masses or ascites, the sacral region for oedema and the legs for ankle oedema, evidence of venous thrombosis, circulatory status and clubbing. While examining the patient in this way, other aspects of the general medical examination should be conducted en route.

Bedside assessment of lung function

Clinical assessment can be made at the bedside of a number of aspects of lung function.
• *Ventilatory capacity* may be assessed by two simple manoeuvres. Firstly, observation and palpation of the lower chest from behind gives an indication of the likely vital capacity and thus of any restrictive defect. The traditional measurement of chest expansion is misleading in this regard. The number that can be attained while counting at one second intervals during a single expiration is also a reasonable indication of vital capacity. Secondly, the patient can be asked to breathe out from a full inspiration as hard and as long as possible. The forced expired time thus measured is normally 3−5 sec. It gives an indication of the forced expiratory volume in one second. Thus, prolongation suggests obstruction and shortening suggests restriction.
• Measurement of the inspiratory time during quiet breathing gives some guide to *ventilatory effort*. Increased effort in response to increased respiratory drive is reflected in a shortening of the inspiratory time to less than 1 sec. On the other hand, decreased respiratory drive is best assessed by the

indices of hypoventilation, namely decreased minute ventilation and/or hypercapnia.

● Other aspects of lung function which may be assessed at the bedside include indices of *gas exchange*. Hypoxaemia and hypercapnia if sufficiently severe give rise to typical, though not specific, clinical features as outlined in Chapter 7 (Respiratory Failure).

4   Lung Function Tests

Introduction

Many respiratory diseases require one or more of the large range of available clinical investigations to clarify the diagnosis, to quantify an abnormality, to follow progress or to guide therapy. The particular measurements or procedures used are determined by the results of the history and physical examination of the patient. The results of the clinical investigations do not logically stand alone but should always be interpreted in the light of the patient's clinical features. The present chapter discusses lung function tests and the next chapter (Chapter 5) imaging, bronchoscopy and other investigations.

Lung function tests have become widely available in major hospitals. Ideally perhaps the broader term, respiratory function, should be used rather than lung function or pulmonary function. As their name indicates, these tests measure physiology, not anatomy or pathology. They cannot, therefore, make diagnoses in most respiratory diseases, since diagnoses are not usually based on function alone. Nevertheless, some diseases do have characteristic patterns of abnormal function, in which case these tests can help diagnosis. Mostly, however, the clinical value of lung function tests is to quantify the defect produced by disease, to follow therapy, to assess fitness for surgery and to explain symptoms such as dyspnoea. Lung function tests are also used in epidemiological surveys of the frequency of certain respiratory disorders and of risk factors.

The intelligent use of lung function tests requires knowledge of their limitations and of the aspect of physiology that a particular test is defining. Although there is a bewildering array of lung function tests potentially available, most information on which clinical decisions are based can be obtained using a limited range of simple tests. The two most commonly used groups of tests are those which measure mechanical function or ventilation and those which measure gas exchange.

Mechanical function

The spirometric measurement of ventilatory capacity provides the most rapid, simple and generally useful assessment of the mechanical properties of the lungs and thoracic cage. Although it is a considerable oversimplification, in practical terms an obstructive defect may be considered to reflect increased airway resistance and a restrictive defect decreased compliance.

Other more sophisticated tests of the mechanical function of the lungs (lung mechanics) include assessment of their static, elastic properties (compliance) and of their dynamic, resistive properties (resistance). By and large, these latter tests are more complex to perform and have been of limited clinical application, though they have been invaluable in enhancing understanding of pulmonary physiology. Body plethysmography is commonly used for these tests, since it permits the rapid and accurate measurement of lung volumes (thoracic gas volumes) at the same time as lung mechanics.

Ventilatory capacity

Ventilatory capacity is measured by having the patient expire maximally into a displacement spirometer or through a calibrated pneumotachograph. The manoeuvre may be performed slowly or with maximum effort. Thus, the vital capacity (VC) may be measured as a slow VC or forced VC (FVC). Normally the VC is similar under both circumstances but in patients with severe airflow limitation, the FVC may be considerably less than the slow VC. This phenomenon has been attributed to airway closure and air trapping due to the generation of high transmural pressure gradients in the presence of narrowed or collapsible airways.

One of the timed components of the FVC is also measured, such as the forced expiratory volume in 1 sec (FEV_1) or the maximum mid-expiratory flow rate (MMEFR). The FEV_1 is the maximum amount of air that can be forcibly expelled in 1 sec and is normally about 75% of the VC. The MMEFR is the average flow rate measured between 25 and 75% of the total expired volume.

The VC gives a simple, robust and reproducible measure of ventilatory capacity or the ability to generate a normal rate and volume of maximum airflow. The VC is reduced in both obstructive and restrictive disorders. In obstruction, the FEV_1 is decreased more than the VC, so that the FEV_1/VC ratio falls (Fig. 4.1). The MMEFR correlates highly with the FEV_1 but is more sensitive to mild obstruction and to abnormalities within small airways. The peak expiratory flow (PEF) may be measured with one of several available peak flowmeters and reflects the flow rate achieved in the first fraction of a second of forced expiration. The PEF measurement is simple enough for field or home use and also correlates well with the FEV_1 (Fig. 4.2).

The acute effect of bronchodilator aerosol on the ventilatory capacity, and in particular on the FEV_1, gives information about the potential reversibility of airways obstruction. If the patient has a history suggestive of airways obstruction but the spirogram is currently normal, an alternative method of assessing lability of airways calibre is to use an inhaled bronchoconstrictor agent, such as methacholine or histamine. Common

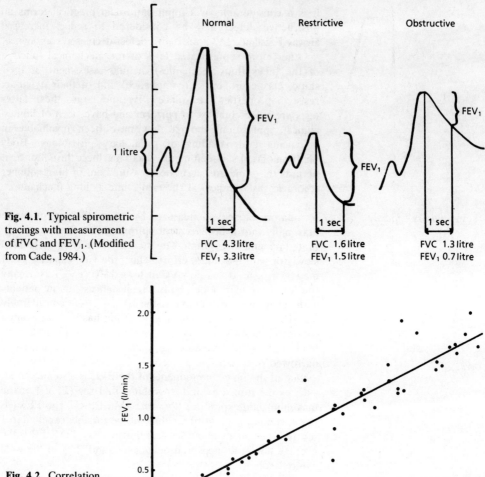

Fig. 4.1. Typical spirometric tracings with measurement of FVC and FEV$_1$. (Modified from Cade, 1984.)

Normal
FEV$_1$
1 litre
1 sec
FVC 4.3 litre
FEV$_1$ 3.3 litre

Restrictive
FEV$_1$
1 sec
FVC 1.6 litre
FEV$_1$ 1.5 litre

Obstructive
FEV$_1$
1 sec
FVC 1.3 litre
FEV$_1$ 0.7 litre

Fig. 4.2. Correlation between spirometry (FEV$_1$) and PEF measured with a Wright Peak Flow Mini-meter (r = 0.89).

FEV$_1$ (l/min)

Peak Expiratory Flow Rate (l/min)

methods of expressing bronchial reactivity are as the percentage change in FEV$_1$ from baseline after one of these manoeuvres, or (for bronchoconstriction) as the dose required to give a standard fall (usually 20%) in FEV$_1$.

The traditional spirogram records volume on the Y-axis against time on the X-axis. If instead the information is expressed as volume on the X-axis plotted against flow on the Y-axis, a flow—volume curve is produced (Fig. 4.3). The slope and shape of the expiratory flow—volume curve has been of particular value in assessing the degree, site and mechanisms of airways obstruction. A complete flow—volume loop may be obtained by recording the same information during inspiration as well as expiration (Fig. 4.4).

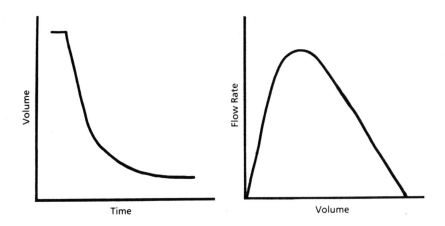

Fig. 4.3. A forced expiratory manoeuvre can be plotted as volume against time (left, traditional spirogram) or as flow against volume (right, flow−volume curve).

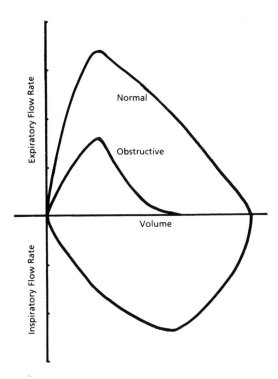

Fig. 4.4. A normal maximal expiratory and inspiratory flow−volume curve. Within this curve is an expiratory maximal flow-volume curve in a patient with airflow obstruction.

The measurement of ventilatory capacity during inspiration, using either the traditional volume−time plot or a flow−volume plot, is useful in detecting airflow limitation due to obstruction of the large extrathoracic airways. In this situation, the inspiratory index (e.g. forced inspiratory volume in 1 sec, FIV_1; maximum mid-inspiratory flow rate, MMIFR) is more

37/*Lung Function Tests*

abnormal than the corresponding expiratory index and their ratio is thus less than 1 (normally, this ratio is 1 or greater).

Compliance

The elastic properties of the lung are described by its pressure—volume relations. The pressure used in this calculation is the transpulmonary pressure, which is the pressure difference between the alveoli and the surface of the lungs. The latter is called intrapleural or intrathoracic pressure and is usually measured in the oesophagus. The alveolar pressure is equal to mouth pressure when there is no airflow. In practice, compliance is measured as the slope of the pressure—volume curve at FRC and is derived from the plot of volume against transpulmonary pressure measured serially during the brief plateaus of no flow which are produced when the subject inspires to TLC or expires from TLC in increments (Fig. 4.5). As previously discussed, the static compliance (or the change in volume of lung per unit of transpulmonary pressure change) depends on a variety of factors which include the amount, arrangement and integrity of the elastic tissue, the surface tension of the alveolar lining fluid and the lung size. Decreased compliance is thus due to stiffer lung tissue, higher surface tension of the alveolar lining fluid or decreased lung volume. Increased compliance is seen in emphysema. The reciprocal of compliance is termed elastance.

Compliance may also be measured dynamically, i.e. during normal breathing, when it is found to be somewhat less than static compliance, particularly if there is non-uniform distribution of mechanical function (i.e. unequal time constants)

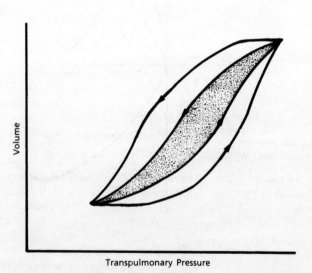

Fig. 4.5. Pressure—volume relationships during maximal inspiration and expiration. The shaded area represents the normal; the outer curve is abnormal, indicating increased work of breathing.

within the lungs. This difference increases as the frequency of breathing increases, a phenomenon referred to as frequency dependence of compliance. This test is difficult to perform reliably but has been shown to be a sensitive index of abnormality of the small airways.

The forces required to overcome the elastic resistance to breathing have to be expended on the chest wall as well as on the lungs. Total thoracic compliance is relevant in that the lungs and chest wall act in concert and the pressure−volume relations applicable clinically, either as a result of respiratory muscle activity or a mechanical ventilator, are those of the entire respiratory system. However, the separate measure of lung compliance gives a purer view of actual pulmonary dysfunction. The chest wall compliance is normally about the same as the lung compliance.

Resistance

The resistive properties of the lung are described by its pressure−flow relations. As for compliance, the pressure involved is also the transpulmonary pressure. Airway resistance is usually measured as the pressure gradient required to generate airflow during quiet breathing. As for compliance, an oesophageal balloon is required to measure intrapleural pressure, while flow is measured with a pneumotachograph. That portion of the transpulmonary pressure required for elastic expansion is subtracted from the total transpulmonary pressure and the remainder is considered to be pressure generating airflow. Other simpler measures of measuring airway resistance include the application of Boyle's law to the changes in pressure and volume obtained when a subject pants through a pneumotachograph while sitting in a body plethysmograph, or the use of forced air oscillations from a sine wave generator (e.g. a loudspeaker) to produce pressure−flow changes at the mouth.

Increased airway resistance is due almost entirely to decreased calibre of the larger airways. This is because the smaller airways contribute little to total resistance and because the non-elastic resistance, such as tissue resistance and inertial forces, are negligible. The reciprocal of resistance is termed conductance and when related to lung size is termed specific conductance.

Work of breathing

The work of breathing is calculated from pressure−volume plots during inspiration and expiration, because the area of such a graph (pressure x volume) has the dimension of work (Fig. 4.5). The area is increased both by decreasing the slope (decreasing compliance) and by the inspiratory to expiratory difference becoming greater (increased resistance).

Ventilation

Total ventilation (minute volume) is usually measured with a spirometer or calibrated flowmeter. Minute volume ($\dot{V}_E$) is divided by the respiratory rate (f) to give the average tidal volume (V_T or TV). The measurement of total ventilation and its components is primarily of value in artificially ventilated patients.

Lung volumes

Lung volumes other than VC and TV may be measured either by gas dilution (e.g. helium) or washout (e.g. nitrogen) or by body plethysmography using Boyle's law. The former methods directly measure FRC and the latter TLC. From knowledge of either FRC or TLC plus spirometric measurements of VC, TV and either inspiratory reserve volume (IRV) or expiratory reserve volume (ERV), all the other subdivisions of the lung volumes can easily be calculated. There may be a discrepancy between the TLC measured by gas dilution or washout methods and that (sometimes called thoracic gas volume, TGV) measured by body plethysmography. The latter gives higher values, particularly in emphysema or in the presence of non-communicating gas spaces, and the difference is a measure of the amount of 'air trapping'. Other than VC, measurements of the other subdivisions of the lung volumes are of limited value in most clinical situations, although they have been extensively applied in research.

Distribution of ventilation

The distribution of ventilation within the lungs is usually measured by analysing the effects on expired gas of a sudden change in the composition of the inspired gas. The change in expired nitrogen can be analysed following a single breath of oxygen (single breath nitrogen test) or during continuous oxygen breathing (nitrogen washout test). Instead of oxygen, the single breath test can also be performed with a tracer gas such as argon or radioactive xenon. An upward sloping expiratory plateau for the single breath test or a prolonged washout indicates poor mixing of the inspiratory gas with gas already present in the lungs and thus maldistribution of ventilation. The terminal part of the expired plateau may show a sudden change in marker gas concentration (Fig. 4.6). The point at which this occurs is thought to coincide with airway closure in certain dependent airways but the closing volume test which is based on this phenomenon has not been clinically useful. Tests of the distribution of ventilation give no direct information about the more important distribution of ventilation in relation to blood flow but since compensatory vascular redistribution can never be ideal, maldistribution of ventilation implies at least some degree of ventilation/blood flow inequality.

Gas exchange

Tests which assess gas exchange include arterial blood gas analysis, measurement of alveolar gas tensions and calculation of indices of ventilation/blood flow matching, and measurements of gas transfer (diffusing capacity).

Arterial blood gas analysis

The measurement of oxygen and carbon dioxide tensions in arterial blood gives direct information on the ability of the lungs to exchange gas between the environment and the blood. Arterial blood gas analysis is the most frequently used test of

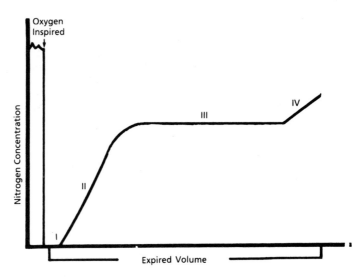

Fig. 4.6. The pattern of expired nitrogen concentration following a single inspirate of oxygen. Phase I represents dead-space gas, phase II mixed dead-space and alveolar gas and phase III alveolar gas. The transition between phase III and a final steep rise (phase IV) indicates airway closure in dependent regions of the lung.

respiratory function, especially in hospital patients, and is the measurement upon which the assessment of respiratory failure is made. It is so important that it is separately considered in Chapter 6.

Alveolar gas tensions and ventilation/blood flow relations

The understanding of gas exchange has been greatly aided by the measurement or calculation of alveolar gas tensions and by the use of simple three compartment conceptual models of the lung. Knowledge of alveolar as well as blood gas tensions is essential for appreciating the magnitude of the driving pressure for gas exchange between the environment and the blood. However, representative alveolar gas is not easily obtained for analysis and 'true' alveolar gas is even difficult to define. Even in health, alveoli empty asynchronously, a process which becomes much more marked in disease. Thus, poorly ventilated areas empty last giving high end-tidal carbon dioxide values, while poorly perfused areas may empty promptly even though they contribute little to gas exchange. In normal lungs, the tracing of the continuous measurement of expired gas such as carbon dioxide reaches a plateau, so that alveolar gas is approximated by an end-tidal sample taken at the end of normal expiration. In abnormal lungs, the tracing is often continuously sloping so that no clear plateau is ever reached and an end-tidal sample is not a reasonable reflection of alveolar gas. Thus, since true alveolar air cannot be readily measured, its composition has to be calculated indirectly. This is done using the concept of 'ideal' alveolar air (Fig. 4.7).

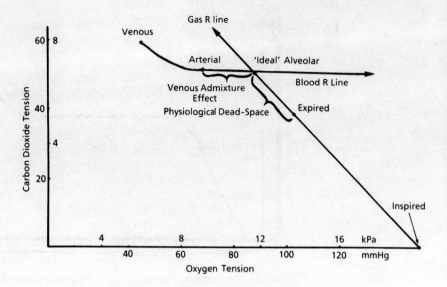

Fig. 4.7. Graphical analysis of gas exchange using the $O_2 : CO_2$ diagram and the concept of 'ideal' alveolar air. Two equations are represented. The alveolar gas equation with a fixed inspired gas composition and gas exchange ratio gives the gas R line; the blood gas exchange equation with a fixed mixed venous blood gas composition and gas exchange ratio gives the blood R line. The point of intersection of the two R lines gives the gas composition of alveolar gas and end-capillary blood in a normal or 'ideal' gas exchanging unit (or in units having the same ventilation/blood flow ratio and the same mixed venous blood, inspired gas and gas exchange ratio). The extent to which the mixed arterial blood gas composition moves from the 'ideal' point along the blood R line and the mixed expired gas composition moves from the 'ideal' point along the gas R line are expressions of ventilation/blood flow inhomogeneity. They are quantitated as venous admixture effect and physiological dead-space, respectively. (Modified from Cade, 1984.)

Using a three compartment model (Chapter 2, Fig. 2.4), the gas exchanging areas within the lung can be divided into:
1 those areas which have increased ventilation in relation to blood flow (and therefore resemble *dead-space* or 'wasted' ventilation and have high V/Q ratios);
2 those areas which have decreased ventilation in relation of blood flow (and therefore resemble *venoarterial shunt* or 'wasted' blood flow and have low V̇/Q̇ ratios); and
3 those areas which have well matched ventilation and blood flow (and have normal V̇/Q̇ ratios).

The areas of relative overventilation (alveolar dead-space) cause an increased disparity between the mixed expired ($P_{E}CO_2$ and mean end-capillary (arterial) carbon dioxide tensions (P_aCO_2). Simultaneous collection and analysis of these samples permits quantitation of the wastefully ventilated areas as the physiologic dead-space to tidal volume ratio (V_D/V_T). This is calculated as:

$$V_D/V_T = \frac{P_aCO_2 - P_{\bar{E}}CO_2}{P_aCO_2}$$

Alveolar or effective ventilation is:

$$\dot{V}_A = \dot{V}_E (1 - V_D/V_T)$$

Conversely, the areas of relative underventilation (venous admixture) cause an increased disparity between the alveolar (P_AO_2) and mean end-capillary (arterial) oxygen tension (P_aO_2). Simultaneous collection and analysis of these samples permits quantitation of the wastefully perfused areas as the ideal alveolar to arterial oxygen tension gradient or as the venoarterial shunt fraction of the cardiac output (Q_s/Q_t) The ideal alveolar oxygen tension is calculated as:

$$P_AO_2 = P_IO_2 - \frac{P_aCO_2}{R}$$

where P_IO_2 is the inspired oxygen tension and R is the respiratory quotient or gas exchange ratio.

The venoarterial shunt is calculated as:

$$\dot{Q}_s/\dot{Q}_t = \frac{C_cO_2 - C_aO_2}{C_cO_2 - C_{\bar{v}}O_2}$$

where C_cO_2, C_aO_2 and $C_{\bar{v}}O_2$ are the contents of oxygen in pulmonary end-capillary, arterial and mixed venous blood.

This three compartment approach to the quantitation of gas exchange abnormalities has been both useful and instructive and is still widely employed. It is, however, a somewhat unreal model when applied to most lung disease in which there is usually a wide spectrum of ventilation/blood flow ratios.

More sophisticated analyses of the distribution of ventilation/blood flow ratios can be made using the measurement of the elimination from the lungs of a range of injected foreign gases. Six inert gases dissolved in saline are infused intravenously and after a steady state has been reached, arterial and expired gas concentrations are measured by sensitive techniques. Since the gases have different solubilities, they partition themselves between blood and air according to the ventilation/blood flow ratio. Calculations may then be derived which describe the continuous distribution of ventilation/blood flow ratios plotted against ventilation or blood flow (Fig. 4.8).

Gas transfer

Gas transfer across the alveolar-capillary membrane is by diffusion, a process which depends on the area, thickness and diffusion coefficient of the membrane, the solubility and size of the molecules being transferred, and the driving pressure and time involved. The alveolar-capillary 'membrane'

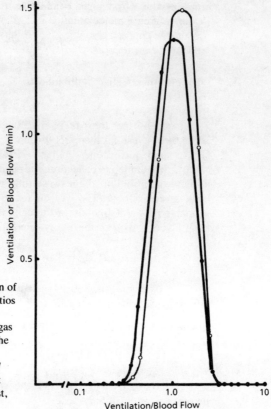

Fig. 4.8. The distribution of ventilation/blood flow ratios in a normal subject as determined by the inert gas technique. The bulk of the lung is ventilated and perfused at a ventilation/ blood flow ratio of about 1.0. (Redrawn from West, 1982.)

comprises the alveolar fluid, alveolar membrane, interstitial fluid, capillary membrane, plasma, red cell membrane and interior of the red cell. For the movement of oxygen and carbon dioxide across the alveolar-capillary membrane, the much greater solubility of carbon dioxide outweighs all other factors. The diffusing capacity is expressed as the volume of gas transferred per unit time per unit of driving pressure.

The diffusing capacity of the lung for oxygen is approximated by that for carbon monoxide, since carbon monoxide also combines with haemoglobin and its rate of diffusion is similar to that of oxygen. The advantage of using carbon monoxide for this purpose is that its mean capillary pressure is virtually zero because of the great affinity of haemoglobin for it, especially at the low concentrations commonly used (less than 0.3%). Thus, during short exposure times this pressure does not actually have to be measured. The only measurements then required are the volume of carbon monoxide taken up per unit time and the other component of the driving pressure, namely the alveolar carbon monoxide tension. Like the other alveolar gas tensions, that for carbon monoxide is not easily and accurately obtained, especially when lung function is abnormal. It is measured in practice using either steady state or single breath methods but in fact, all measurements of diffusing capacity reflect the effective surface area for gas exchange and are thus influenced more by ventilation/blood flow relations than by diffusion itself. A simple and rapid method of assessing gas transfer is to measure the fractional carbon monoxide uptake (FCO) instead of the more formal and complex diffusing capacity ($D_L CO$). The FCO is the proportional extraction of carbon monoxide during a period of steady state, quiet breathing.

The diffusing capacity is of use as a sensitive index of the degree of abnormality of the fine structure of the lung. However, it should be appreciated that abnormalities of the diffusing capacity do not necessarily imply a shrunken or thickened membrane. Indeed, it is doubtful if reduction of the diffusing properties of the alveolar-capillary membrane (in contrast to reduction in its surface area) is ever an important clinical cause of defective oxygen transfer. It is certainly much less important than disturbance of ventilation/blood flow ratios.

Pulmonary blood flow

Pulmonary blood flow is usually considered part of circulatory physiology. However, certain of its features are appropriate to discuss here, since both the volume and distribution of blood flow must be matched to that of ventilation and to the metabolic needs of the body for the lungs to function adequately. Although the volume of ventilation is determined by respiratory factors, the volume of pulmonary blood flow is determined chiefly by the extrapulmonary mechanisms that control cardiac output. The distribution of pulmonary blood flow, however, is determined by pulmonary mechanisms, as previously discussed.

The volume of pulmonary blood flow, or cardiac output (C.O.), is most commonly measured nowadays by thermodilution, a variant of the indicator dilution technique previously used with dye. The measurement of cardiac output and of pulmonary haemodynamics has become widely available in recent years since the introduction of balloon-tipped, flow-directed (Swan-Ganz) catheters. The catheter is usually inserted percutaneously into a large vein (internal jugular, subclavian, median cubital, femoral) and advanced through the right heart into the pulmonary artery where it finally wedges in a peripheral vessel. The pressures measured in turn are right atrial (RA), right ventricular (RV), pulmonary arterial (PA) and finally, the pulmonary artery wedge (PAW, or pulmonary capillary wedge, PCW) pressures (Fig. 4.9). The normal PA pressures are only about one-fifth of the systemic arterial pressures and the pulmonary vasculature is thus a high-volume, low-pressure system. The pulmonary vascular resistance (PVR) is calculated as

$$PVR = \frac{\text{Mean PAP} - \text{PAWP}}{\text{C.O.}}$$

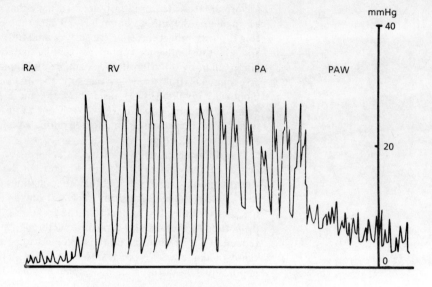

Fig. 4.9. Pressure tracings obtained during progressive catheterization of the right atrium (RA), right ventricle (RV) and pulmonary artery (PA) until the catheter is wedged in a distal pulmonary artery (PAW).

The pulmonary vascular resistance is normally about one-tenth of the systemic vascular resistance and on exercise falls even lower due to pulmonary vasodilatation and the opening of vessels normally closed at rest.

Although global pulmonary blood flow (cardiac output) and pulmonary haemodynamics are readily measured, the distribution of blood flow within the lungs is not accessible to routine assessment in man in vivo, apart from isotopic techniques which indicate local changes and physiological methods which indicate overall changes in distribution.

Blood gas transport

Blood gas transport is assessed by measuring the separate components of oxygen and carbon dioxide carriage in the blood. For example, for oxygen the individual components are respiratory (oxygen saturation), haematological (haemoglobin) and circulatory (cardiac output). The details of blood gas transport are considered in Chapter 6 (Blood Gas Analysis).

Control of ventilation

The control of ventilation may be measured by a number of methods. Most have used the ventilatory response to carbon dioxide which may be performed by a simple rebreathing technique. The slope of the relation between ventilation and the carbon dioxide level (V_E/P_{CO_2}) is an index primarily of the sensitivity of the central chemoreceptors (Fig. 4.10). A similar technique may be employed to measure the ventilatory

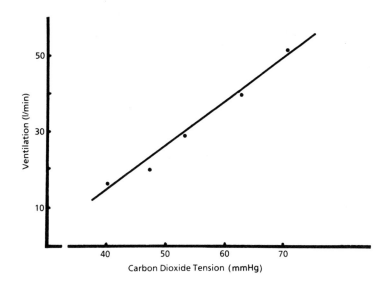

Fig. 4.10. Increase in ventilation with increasing inspired carbon dioxide tension. The shape of the relationship expresses the ventilatory response to carbon dioxide. Data were obtained during a period of rebreathing.

response to hypoxia and thus test primarily the sensitivity of the peripheral chemoreceptors.

One of the chief limitations of measuring the ventilatory response to carbon dioxide in patients with lung disease is that it cannot distinguish between those patients with a decreased response because of a decreased respiratory drive and those patients with a decreased response because of an increased workload. To measure the output of the respiratory centre independently of the mechanical load, simple tests have been developed based on changes in pressure at the mouth during transient occlusion of the airway in early inspiration. These tests are truer reflections of ventilatory drive.

Exercise

Exercise is a valuable manoeuvre with which to uncover information about lung dysfunction which may be well compensated at rest. In other words, it evaluates the amount of functional respiratory reserve which may sometimes be hard to assess, especially early in the course of disease. In addition, exercise helps objectively to quantify the degree of dyspnoea and in some conditions it may also be of specific diagnostic help, such as in exercise-induced asthma, psychogenic dyspnoea, myocardial ischaemia, peripheral vascular disease and unfitness. Exercise stresses the cardiovascular, metabolic and psychological as well as respiratory functions of the body in an integrated and quantifiable manner and is 'physiological' in that in reproduces in the laboratory much of the stress of daily life.

The responses during exercise are most easily studied on a bicycle ergometer, although a treadmill may also be used. The exercise test may be conducted at various levels of complexity. In its simplest form, ventilation, heart rate and ECG are continuously recorded during progressive, multi-stage exercise until maximum tolerance or target heart rate or power output is reached. Oxygen consumption and carbon dioxide production may be measured. At the next level of complexity, a steady state of submaximal exercise of about one-third and two-thirds maximum is maintained, while end-tidal and mixed venous (rebreathing) carbon dioxide tensions are also measured. Arterial blood gas analysis, blood lactate estimation and right heart catheterization may be included in a comprehensive exercise assessment. In practice, most information is obtained with the simpler forms of testing.

Nomograms for predicted values of the different parameters at various exercise levels are readily available and should be consulted when interpreting the results of exercise tests. If spirometry is abnormal and especially if airways obstruction is present, the predicted maximum ventilation may be estimated by multiplying the FEV_1 by 35. When dyspnoea is due primarily to respiratory disease, ventilation tends to be greater than normal throughout the exercise test and reaches its maximum at levels of power output lower than normal. Hypoxaemia and possibly hypercapnia may also occur during exercise in patients with respiratory disease. When dyspnoea is due primarily to cardiac disease, the heart rate tends to be greater than normal throughout the exercise test and reaches its maximum at levels of power output lower than normal. Maximum ventilation is not reached, indicating that there is no respiratory limitation. Since the heart rate at a given power output or oxygen consumption is excessive and since cardiac output bears a linear relation to oxygen consumption, it follows that the normal increase in stroke volume has been impaired.

Regional lung function

Regional lung function studies have generally been of physiological interest rather than of direct clinical application. However, in some clinical situations, it can be useful to have an assessment of regional as well as global function, particularly when there is severe localized disease and, for example, when thoracic surgery is contemplated. Bronchospirometry using differential bronchial catheterization permits the collection of air separately from each lung. Calculations may then be made not only of ventilation but also of lung volumes and gas exchange data for each lung. This technique has been little used in recent years, although methods of differential sampling from different lobes or segments of the lung have been reintroduced using the fibreoptic bronchoscope and mass spectrometry.

The commonest methods of assessing regional lung function have used radioactive isotopes. When a labelled gas (e.g. 133-

Table 4.1. Normal values for lung function tests

Mechanical function		
vital capacity (VC)	5.0	l
total lung capacity (TLC)	7.0	l
residual volume (RV)	2.0	l
functional residual capacity (FRC)	3.3	l
RV/TLC	29	%
forced expired volume in one second (FEV_1)	4.0	l
maximal mid-expiratory flow rate (MMEFR)	3.5	l/sec
peak expiratory flow rate (PEF, PFR)	600	l/sec
maximal inspiratory pressure at FRC (MIP)	80	mmHg
maximal expiratory pressure at TLC (MEP)	130	mmHg
static compliance ($C_L$stat)	0.25	l/cmH$_2$O
airway resistance (R_{aw})	0.2	cmH$_2$O/l/sec

Ventilation		
minute ventilation ($\dot{V}_I$ or $\dot{V}_E$)	7.0	l/min
tidal volume (V_T)	550	ml
frequency (f)	12	/min
alveolar ventilation ($\dot{V}_A$)	4.8	l/min

Arterial blood		
oxygen saturation (S_aO_2)	>95	%
oxygen tension (P_aO_2)		
(breathing air at sea level)	85–100	mmHg
	11–13	kPa
(breathing 100% oxygen)	>600	mmHg
	>80	kPa
carbon dioxide tension (P_aCO_2)	35–44	mmHg
	4.8–5.8	kPa
pH	7.36–7.44	
hydrogen ion concentration	40	nmol/l

Gas exchange		
gas exchange ratio (R)	0.75–0.9	
oxygen consumption ($\dot{V}O_2$)	240	ml/min
carbon dioxide production ($\dot{V}CO_2$)	185	ml/min
alveolar-arterial oxygen tension gradient		
($A-aPO_2$) (breathing air at sea level)	<15	mmHg
	<2	kPa
venous admixture ($\dot{Q}_{va}/\dot{Q}_t$)	7	%
right-to-left shunt ($\dot{Q}_s/\dot{Q}_t$)	3	%
diffusing capacity for carbon monoxide		
single breath technique (D_LCO SB)	25–40	ml/min/mmHg
steady state technique (D_LCO SS)	15–25	ml/min/mmHg
fractional carbon monoxide uptake (FCO)		
(at 10 l/min)	35–45	%

Respiratory control		
ventilatory response to hypercapnia		
($\triangle\dot{V}_E/\triangle PCO_2$)	2.5	l/min/mmHg
ventilatory response to hypoxia ($\triangle\dot{V}_E/\triangle S_aO_2$)	−0.75	l/min/%
mouth occlusion pressure at rest ($P_{0.1}$)	2.1±0.7	cmH$_2$O

Exercise
(see Chapter 2, Table 2.1)

xenon) is inhaled, regions of the lung may be counted externally with scintillation counters or the whole lung with a gamma camera, and expired gas can be counted at the mouth. Xenon is an insoluble gas so that it remains confined to the air spaces when inhaled and is almost entirely evolved into the lungs when injected intravenously. When xenon is rebreathed from an appropriate circuit until the counts are stable, its local concentration reflects local lung volume. When a single large breath of xenon is taken, the counts reflect local ventilation. When xenon is injected as an intravenous bolus, the counts reflect local blood flow (provided there is some local aeration to receive the evolved gas). Thus, regional ventilation, blood flow and volume can be quickly and simply assessed.

A less subtle but very widely used technique which permits assessment of regional lung perfusion is to scan the lungs after the intravenous injection of labelled particles, such as ^{99m}Tc-labelled albumin macro-aggregates or microspheres. About 300 000 particles of about 50 μm in size are injected and they impact in the pulmonary arterioles (less than 1 in 1000 vessels are temporarily occluded) producing regional radioactivity proportional to the local blood flow. This technique has chiefly been applied in the assessment of pulmonary thromboembolism.

Normal values

The average values for lung function tests in a healthy, resting, adult male of weight 70 kg and height 175 cm are shown in Table 4.1. Some indices have a considerable normal range and vary with sex, age and height.

Imaging, Bronchoscopy and Other Investigations

Imaging	Bronchoscopy
Chest X-ray	Other endoscopy
Tomography	Biopsy
Fluoroscopy	Microbiology
Bronchography	Cytology
Angiography	Skin tests
Radionuclide scanning	Electrocardiogram
Ultrasonography	Haematology
Computed tomography	Biochemistry
	Serology

Imaging

Chest X-ray

The chest X-ray has long been an integral part of initial respiratory evaluation. It complements physical examination in so many important ways that it is often best regarded as an extension of the physical examination itself. The chest X-ray is interpreted much more profitably in the light of the patient's clinical features. Conversely, many conditions (e.g. cavitation) are much better elucidated by chest X-ray than by even the most meticulous physical examination. Thus, the integrated findings from the combination of history, physical examination and plain chest X-ray are the mainstay of respiratory evaluation in almost all situations.

In addition, routine chest X-rays are performed in many people (e.g. patients on admission to hospital, normal subject screening) in whom a clinical respiratory assessment has not previously been made. Should the X-ray prove abnormal, the usual sequence of clinical and radiological assessment is reversed but the end result is similar.

The *standard chest X-ray* consists of a posteroanterior (PA) film taken from about 2m with the plate against the front of the chest. This projection minimizes the divergence of X-rays which would cause the heart to appear larger than its true size. In patients confined to bed, an anteroposterior (AP) film is taken with a mobile machine and the plate against the back of the chest. There are many practical and technical difficulties with such portable techniques and in addition, cardiac size can be more difficult to assess. To localize a lesion seen on the plain film, an appropriate lateral X-ray is required. The routine views for plain chest X-ray examination are thus usually PA and left lateral.

The chest X-ray should be examined according to an ordered sequence:

1 An optimally exposed film should have the density and penetration set so that the intervertebral disc spaces are just visible behind the heart.

2 Proper positioning of the patient excludes rotation and

this is checked by noting that the medial ends of each clavicle are equidistant from the spine.

3 The lung fields are subdivided into upper, middle and lower zones on each side. Each zone is carefully examined and compared with other zones.

4 Both hila are checked for position and for masses. Abnormal hilar position is usually due to pulmonary collapse with resultant hilar deviation in that direction. Bilateral hilar enlargement usually indicates lymphadenopathy or pulmonary artery dilatation. Unilateral hilar enlargement is suggestive of tumour.

5 The heart is examined for size and shape, and retrocardiac lesions (e.g. collapsed left lower lobe) should be carefully sought.

6 The upper mediastinum is viewed for masses (retrosternal thyroid, lymphadenopathy, aortic aneurysm) and for the tracheal position and shape.

7 The bony cage is examined for deformity, osteolytic lesions or rib notching from coarctation of the aorta.

8 The hemidiaphragm and costophrenic and cardiophrenic angles are checked. Normally the right hemidiaphragm is 1−2 cm higher than the left.

9 The extrathoracic soft tissues, including the breasts, should be examined for contour, foreign body, calcification and subcutaneous emphysema.

10 Finally, any previous films should always be obtained for comparison.

Special views are sometimes required to clarify lesions difficult to see on routine films. Common supplementary projections include lordotic, lateral decubitus and oblique, and increased penetration is sometimes used. A lordotic or apical projection raises the clavicles above the lung fields and improves the views of the apices. A lateral decubitus film, with the affected side uppermost, helps determine whether suspected fluid is lying free in the pleural space. Slightly oblique views (20%) help clarify paravertebral lesions, pleural thickening and localized calcification, and more oblique views (60%) better define the cardiac valves and aorta. Penetrated views are useful for examining denser structures, such as those in the mediastinum or spine, or those obscured by overlying tissues.

Tomography

Tomography is a radiological technique for examining, in fine detail, a section of lung at a particular depth. It is of chief value in elucidating the nature of localized lesions, particularly nodules, cavities or arteriovenous malformations.

Fluoroscopy

Fluoroscopy, or radiological screening, permits the continuous examination of the lungs, diaphragm and heart during normal cardiorespiratory movement. An image intensifier is used for the purpose. This once popular technique is much less used nowadays, although its use has increased again recently as an aid to accurate positioning of the fibreoptic bronchoscope and forceps for transbronchial lung biopsy. Traditional fluoroscopy is chiefly of value in examining diaphragmatic movement.

Bronchography

Bronchography defines the anatomy of the tracheobronchial tree following the instillation of liquid contrast medium. This technique has also fallen into substantial disuse in recent times, because it is unpleasant for the patient and because for many purposes it has been superseded by fibreoptic bronchoscopy. Its chief value has been, and to some extent still remains, in the elucidation of bronchiectasis (particularly if surgery is contemplated) and in some cases of haemoptysis.

Angiography

Angiography defines the anatomy of the pulmonary vascular tree following the injection into the pulmonary artery of contrast medium. More proximal injection does not usually provide optimal angiographic quality, although this usual limitation has changed dramatically with the recent advent of *digital subtraction angiography*. More distal injection provides selective angiography in greater detail.

The procedure is performed using an image intensifier and the angiograms are taken either with a rapid film changer or with cinematography. Pulmonary haemodynamics can also be readily measured during the procedure. Pulmonary angiography is performed mainly for the definitive diagnosis of pulmonary embolism, particularly when the issue is equivocal despite radionuclide lung scanning. The occasional pulmonary angiogram which used to be performed for evaluation of arteriovenous malformations or of hilar masses would nowadays be superseded by computed tomography. Pulmonary angiography is an invasive procedure and is not performed with great frequency in most institutions, although it has retained its place as the yardstick for the diagnosis of pulmonary embolism during life.

Radionuclide scanning

Radionuclide scanning of the lungs, particularly perfusion scanning, is widely available and has been the mainstay of routine objective investigation of pulmonary thromboembolism for many years.

● *Perfusion lung scanning* is performed on the supine subject with a gamma camera or a rectilinear scanner following the intravenous injection of suitable labelled particles, such as ^{99m}Tc-labelled albumin macro-aggregates or microspheres. As these particles impact in the pulmonary arterioles, regional radioactivity is proportional to the regional blood flow. Reduced pulmonary blood flow is easily recognized as an area of decreased radioactivity on the scan. Thus, the chief indication for such scans is suspected pulmonary vascular occlusion.

● *Ventilation lung scanning* is performed following the inhalation of a gas mixture, usually containing a small amount of 133-xenon. Reduced pulmonary ventilation is thus apparent as an area of decreased radioactivity on the scan. The main application of ventilation lung scanning is in clarifying topographical ventilation/blood flow relations is cases of suspected pulmonary embolism. For example, some perfusion defects may be secondary to local lung disease, in which case there is associated poor local ventilation; others may be due to primary vascular obstruction, in which case local ventilation remains relatively normal.

• *Gallium lung scanning* following the intravenous injection two to three days previously of 67-gallium citrate can indicate areas of increased uptake by concentrations of leucocytes or neoplastic cells. Although relatively non-specific, gallium scanning has some value in the assessment of activity in inflammatory conditions such as sarcoidosis, in detecting occult pulmonary infection in septicaemic patients and in localizing sites of primary lung tumours or lymphoma.

Ultrasonography

Ultrasonography is an imaging technique that has been in well established clinical use for many years, particularly for cardiac and abdominal examination. It has, however, not yet found a useful place in the investigation of pulmonary disorders.

Computed tomography

Computed tomography (CT scanning) is a recently introduced imaging technique which has revolutionized the radiological investigation of lesions in many parts of the body, particularly in the head, where it was first applied, but more recently in other areas, such as the chest. A cross-sectional slice of the body is examined by having the X-ray source and detector rotate about the body at that site. Serial slices are examined and the data are computer-processed for subsequent display in the form of anatomical maps of tissue of varying radiodensity. Enhancement of the image can be obtained by simultaneous injection of contrast medium intravenously to outline vascular structures more densely.

CT scanning is sophisticated and expensive, and thus not available outside major centres. However, it is a sensitive technique for examining many lung nodules, pleural lesions, aortic aneurysms, and particularly mediastinal spread of carcinoma. Together with fibreoptic bronchoscopy it has superseded many older radiological techniques, though its precise role is still being clarified.

Newer imaging techniques such as *magnetic resonance imaging* (MRI or nuclear magnetic resonance NMR) and *positron emission tomography* (PET) are presently being evaluated. Although MRI appears to have promising widespread application, including examination of the chest, PET has so far been chiefly applied to the analysis of the biochemical behaviour of the brain.

Bronchoscopy

Bronchoscopy is an essential aid in respiratory medicine. It permits direct viewing of the tracheobronchial tree and thus contributes both to diagnosis and management in many pulmonary disorders. Nowadays, most examinations are performed with a flexible, fibreoptic bronchoscope. This is a rather expensive and somewhat delicate instrument but it enables the whole of the tracheobronchial tree to be inspected, at least as far as the subsegmental bronchi. It is usually passed transnasally under local anaesthesia and causes minimal patient discomfort. It can also be passed via an endotracheal or tracheostomy tube, even in a mechanically ventilated patient. A fine brush or biopsy forceps can be passed down the special channel in the bronchoscope for tissue sampling. Secretions can also be directly aspirated for cytology or microbiological examination via the same channel, if necessary following saline lavage. The main disadvantages of fibreoptic bronchoscopy are that, because of the fine sampling channel, biopsy specimens are very small, suction is too limited to control major haemorrhage and it is unsuitable for the removal of most foreign bodies. The older, rigid bronchoscope is still required for the latter two situations.

The chief indications for bronchoscopy are suspicion of carcinoma, bronchial obstruction, haemoptysis, collection of secretions or lavage fluid for microbiological or cytological examination, removal of foreign body or secretions (bronchial toilet), bronchial trauma and biopsy of intraluminal or diffuse lung lesions. Although the technique is very safe, particular care should be exercised in patients with arrhythmias, respiratory failure, severe obstruction and in the biopsy of a possible bronchial adenoma. The main complications are bleeding or pneumothorax which may follow transbronchial biopsy but these are rarely life-threatening.

Other endoscopy

Other pulmonary endoscopic procedures include mediastinoscopy and thoracoscopy.
• *Mediastinoscopy* involves the passage of an instrument into the anterior mediastinum via a small incision, usually in the suprasternal notch. Mediastinal nodes as far as the carina may be inspected and biopsied. This technique has greatly reduced the need for exploratory thoracotomy in bronchogenic carcinoma, although, in turn, it is being at least partly superseded by CT scanning.
• *Thoracoscopy* with visual inspection of the pleural space and appropriate biopsy can be useful when pleural nodules are present.

Biopsy

Biopsy via a bronchoscope may be either *endobronchial* or *transbronchial*. The former refers to the biopsy of endobronchial lesions directly visible. The latter refers to the biopsy of lesions, either solid or diffuse, beyond the view of the bronchoscope. For solid lesions, the biopsy forceps are best guided under fluoroscopic control. For diffuse disease, the forceps are pushed beyond the field of view and through the bronchial wall, where multiple samples are taken, preferably from those areas of lung shown radiologically to be most affected.

55/*Imaging, Bronchoscopy and Other Investigations*

• *Open lung biopsy* requires a small though formal thoracotomy and nowadays is usually performed only when transbronchial biopsy has failed to yield a diagnostic result. Its chief value is in diffuse lung disease and its main advantage is in obtaining samples of adequate size for histological examination, again preferably from an area of the lung known to be radiologically involved and inspected by the surgeon at operation.

• *Percutaneous needle aspiration biospy* may be used for discrete peripheral lesions. This form of biopsy is usually performed with a long aspirating needle guided to the lesion fluoroscopically or under CT control. Cellular fragments so obtained are examined cytologically and microbiologically. The technique has been used mainly for the diagnosis of malignancy or of pulmonary infections. Older percutaneous techniques involving the use of a high-speed drill or a trephine needle are rarely used now.

• *Pleural biopsy* is easily performed under local anaesthesia using a biopsy punch. Its chief application is in the diagnosis of malignancy or tuberculosis involving the parietal pleura and associated with a pleural effusion. It is usually combined with pleural aspiration.

Microbiology

Microbiological examination of tracheobronchial secretions is a key element in the diagnosis of respiratory infections. These secretions are most commonly obtained as expectorated sputum, but may also be collected from direct tracheobronchial suction with a sterile catheter in intubated patients, from transtracheal aspiration with a fine needle and catheter, from bronchial washings during bronchoscopy and sometimes from gastric lavage. Saliva and upper respiratory tract secretions are completely inappropriate for microbiological examination. Gross inspection of the sputum is followed by microscopic screening of a Gram-stained smear. Excessive numbers of squamous cells indicate a predominantly upper respiratory tract origin and the specimen should not be processed further. A satisfactory sputum sample instead contains numerous alveolar macrophages. Microscopy may reveal the presence of pus cells as well as micro-organisms, and sometimes eosinophils, Charcot–Leyden crystals, Curschmann's spirals, or particles (e.g. asbestos bodies). Sputum culture is then performed, both for definitive diagnosis of pathogenic bacteria and for antibiotic sensitivity testing. Bronchial brushings, biopsy material and pleural fluid are also examined microbiologically in a similar way.

Cytology

Cytological examination of sputum, bronchial washings and pleural fluid for malignant cells is a valuable diagnostic method in experienced hands.

Skin tests

Skin tests are useful in assessing the immunological response of patients with a variety of respiratory disorders. The best known is the tuberculin or Mantoux test for tuberculosis. Reagents are also available for skin testing for a variety of other bacterial, fungal and protozoal respiratory pathogens. Skin prick testing for respiratory allergens, such as house dust mite, grasses, pollens and moulds, is a useful adjunct in the diagnosis of allergic respiratory disorders.

Electrocardiogram

The electrocardiogram (ECG) provides evidence of right heart strain in severe respiratory disease, such as advanced chronic airways obstruction, severe pulmonary fibrosis or major pulmonary embolism. ECG demonstration of left heart disease is relevant in cases of acute pulmonary oedema.

Haematology

Haematological examination is required to demonstrate the presence of polycythaemia in chronic hypoxaemia, anaemia in some cases of dyspnoea, leucocytosis in respiratory infections, eosinophilia in hypersensitivity disorders, and disseminated intravascular coagulation in some severely ill patients with the adult respiratory distress syndrome.

Biochemistry

Biochemical studies are useful in many cases of respiratory disease. Some examples include indices of hepatic and renal dysfunction in patients with multisystem disease, endocrine abnormalities in lung carcinoma, sweat sodium concentration in cystic fibrosis, and serum levels of α_1-antitrypsin in emphysema, calcium in sarcoidosis and metastatic carcinoma, immunoglobulins in multiple myeloma, 5-hydroxy indole acetic acid in carcinoid, and angiotensin converting enzyme in sarcoidosis.

Serology

Serology is of diagnostic value in two situations. Firstly, tests for systemic lupus erythematosus, rheumatoid arthritis and autoimmune antigens are indicated when respiratory involvement is suspected in association with systemic disease, the nature of which may not always be clear. Secondly, raised titres of specific antibody occur in many respiratory infections, particularly atypical ones, such as those due to viruses, mycoplasma and legionella.

6   Blood Gas Analysis

Introduction

Arterial blood gas analysis gives direct information on the ability of the lungs to exchange oxygen and carbon dioxide between the environment and the blood, and on the acid–base state of the body as a whole. It is the most frequently used test of respiratory function, especially in hospitalized patients, both because of the wide availability of blood gas analysers and because of its importance, since it is the measurement upon which the assessment of respiratory failure is made.

Arterial oxygen tension

The arterial oxygen tension (P_aO_2) gives several types of information. Firstly, it indicates the efficiency of oxygenation by the lungs and is therefore an index of lung function. Secondly, it is a major component of blood oxygen transport and is therefore an index of the adequacy of oxygen delivery. Thirdly, when the measurement of oxygen tension in arterial blood is combined with its measurement in (mixed) venous blood, the oxygen gradient across the tissues can be calculated and thus a global estimate of circulatory function can be made.

An index of lung function

The assessment of the gas exchange function of the lungs from knowledge of the arterial oxygen tension clearly requires that the inspired oxygen concentration is also known. For example, an arterial oxygen tension of 100 mmHg has quite different implications for lung function if the subject is breathing air (in which case gas exchange is normal) or 100% oxygen (in which case gas exchange is grossly abnormal).

This index of lung function is quantified as the gradient of oxygen tension between the alveoli and pulmonary venous (= arterial) blood, usually called the alveolar-arterial oxygen tension gradient (or A-a difference in PO_2). This is calculated from the ideal alveolar air equation (see Chapter 4).

$$P_AO_2 = P_IO_2 - P_ACO_2 \left(F_IO_2 + \frac{1 - F_IO_2}{R} \right)$$

As previously shown, this equation is generally used in its abbreviated form:

$$P_AO_2 = P_IO_2 - \frac{P_aCO_2}{R}$$

For example, in a normal subject breathing air:

$$P_{A}O_2 = 150 \text{ mmHg} - \frac{40 \text{ mmHg}}{0.8} = 100 \text{ mmHg}$$

If in this same subject the arterial Po_2 is 90 mmHg, the alveolar-arterial oxyen tension difference is 10 mmHg (normal is less than 15 mmHg or less than 10% of the P_1O_2 for all levels of inspired oxygen). Note that in these (and other) calculations the alveolar carbon dioxide tension ($P_{A}CO_2$) has been replaced by the arterial carbon dioxide tension ($P_{a}CO_2$). This a reasonable approximation as it introduces only a small error into the calculations and, moreover, the $P_{a}CO_2$ is much more easily measured.

<table>
<tr><td>An index of tissue
oxygenation</td><td>

The assessment of tissue oxygen delivery requires knowledge of the three individual components of blood oxygen transport, viz. respiratory (oxygen saturation), haematological (haemoglobin) and circulatory (cardiac output).

</td></tr>
</table>

An index of tissue oxygenation

The assessment of tissue oxygen delivery requires knowledge of the three individual components of blood oxygen transport, viz. respiratory (oxygen saturation), haematological (haemoglobin) and circulatory (cardiac output).

The arterial oxygen tension itself is only an indirect reflection of the amount of oxygen carried in the blood. This in turn is related rather to the *oxygen saturation* or proportional saturation of haemoglobin with oxygen. The relation between oxygen saturation and tension is given by the oxygen dissociation curve, previously discussed in Chapter 2. The oxygen saturation may be directly measured, or may be calculated from the measurement of oxygen tension and the known oxygen dissociation curve.

The actual amount of oxygen carried in the blood (or *oxygen content*) is approximately equal to haemoglobin × saturation × 1.39*, since most of the oxygen in the blood is bound to haemoglobin. However, a small amount of oxygen is directly dissolved in blood (0.3 ml O_2/100 ml blood/100 mmHg pressure). Thus, the arterial oxygen content is normally about 20 ml O_2/100 ml blood (15 × 97% × 1.39 + 0.3). The arterial oxygen content may be calculated in this way or may be directly measured.

If the inspired air is enriched with oxygen, little extra oxygen is normally carried in the blood, because even during air breathing haemoglobin is almost fully saturated with oxygen. The dissolved oxygen, of course, increases linearly as the oxygen tension increases. Thus, if the subject breathes 100% oxygen instead of air and the arterial oxygen tension increases from 100 mmHg to, say, 640 mmHg, the arterial oxygen content would increase by only 10% to about 23 ml O_2/100 ml blood [(15 × 100% × 1.39) + (0.3 × 6.4)].

The rate of oxygen delivered to the tissues is calculated by multiplying the arterial oxygen content by the cardiac output.

*1.39 is the factor currently used in this calculation since 1g of haemoglobin fully saturated with oxygen carries 1.39 ml O_2. A figure of 1.34 was more commonly used in the past but did not take account of common haemoglobin impurities.

Thus, the normal *oxygen delivery* (oxygen transport, oxygen supply or oxygen availability) is approximately equal to 1000 ml O_2/min (20 ml O_2/100 ml blood $\times$ 5 l/min = 1000 ml O_2/min). Of this, about 25% is extracted (utilized or consumed) by the tissues and the remainder returns in the venous blood. Oxygen uptake by the lungs must equal oxygen consumption by the tissues and this is approximately 250 ml/min in the resting state.

Finally, it should be noted that the position of the oxygen dissociation curve is altered by a number of factors, as discussed in Chapter 2. For example, an increase in carbon dioxide shifts the curve to the right (Bohr effect), facilitating the unloading of oxygen in the tissues. A shift in the oxygen dissociation curve (change in affinity of haemoglobin for oxygen) can thus affect oxygen availability in the tissues, even if oxygen transport is unchanged.

A global estimate of circulatory function

When mixed venous as well as arterial oxygen tensions are known, circulatory function can be assessed. This is because the arteriovenous oxygen content difference is determined by the balance between oxygen consumption and cardiac output (the Fick equation). For example, a higher oxygen consumption or a lower cardiac output gives a lower mixed venous oxygen tension, and vice versa. The equation is thus:

$$\text{C.O.} = \frac{\dot{V}_{O_2}}{C_aO_2 - C_{\bar{v}}O_2}$$

If cardiac output is directly measured (e.g. by thermodilution), oxygen consumption can be exactly calculated. Alternatively, oxygen consumption itself may be directly measured but this is not an easy technique.

Since oxygen consumption is determined by the metabolic activity of the body and is normally about 250 ml/min at rest, the cardiac output (normally about 5 l/min) is inversely proportional to the arteriovenous oxygen content difference (normally about 5 ml O_2/100 ml blood). If lung function and oxygen consumption remain unchanged, cardiac output becomes inversely proportional to mixed venous oxygen content (or saturation) — a valuable relation since the continuous measurement of mixed venous oxygen saturatioin has become a practical clinical technique in recent years.

Looked at in a more comprehensive way and transposing the Fick equation:

$$C_{\bar{v}}O_2 = C_aO_2 - \frac{\dot{V}_{O_2}}{\text{C.O.}}$$

This may be paraphrased as:

$$S_{\bar{v}}O_2 = \text{Lungs} - \frac{\text{Metabolism}}{\text{Heart} \times \text{Hb}}$$

Thus, mixed venous oxygen saturation gives in a single index the balance between cardiac function, respiratory function and body metabolism. For example, if mixed venous oxygen saturation is normal (about 75%), neither cardiac nor respiratory function can be abnormal; if mixed venous oxygen saturation is increased, cardiac output must be increased in relation to metabolic needs; if mixed venous oxygen saturation is decreased, multiple respiratory, cardiac and/or metabolic reasons may apply.

Arterial carbon dioxide tension

The arterial carbon dioxide tension (P_aCO_2) gives information about the level of ventilation. For a number of reasons, including greater solubility and the influence of oxygenation on carbon dioxide−haemoglobin equilibrium, the arterial carbon dioxide tension is less affected by internal derangements in pulmonary gas exchange than is the arterial oxygen tension (Fig. 6.1). The arterial carbon dioxide tension is thus not a useful index of lung function (though it is influenced by gross disturbances in lung function). The same considerations apply to carbon dioxide as to oxygen in relation to gradients across the tissues. However, carbon dioxide contents (as opposed to tensions) are not so easily measured or calculated

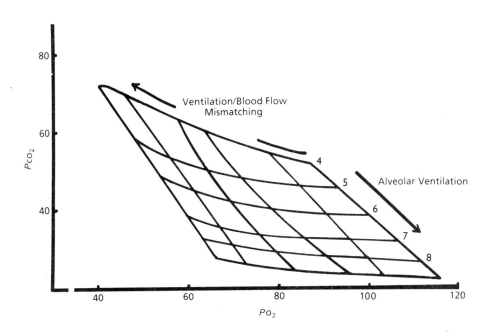

Fig. 6.1. The influence of increasing ventilation/blood flow mismatching and ventilation on arterial blood gas tensions. Note that for any given level of ventilation, worsening ventilation/blood flow relationships cause considerable reduction of oxygenation but only modest elevation of the carbon dioxide level. Data were derived from multicompartment model analysis.

as those for oxygen, so that the oxygen-derived indices are usually used for estimates of global circulatory function.

Since the body's entire load of carbon dioxide produced from metabolic processes is cleared by the lungs, the arterial carbon dioxide tension (strictly the alveolar carbon dioxide tension) gives a direct estimate of the level of ventilation in relation to metabolism. Thus, the alveolar ventilation equation is:

$$P_a\text{co}_2 \propto \frac{\dot{V}\text{co}_2}{\dot{V}_A} = 0.863\frac{\dot{V}\text{co}_2}{\dot{V}_A}$$

where the normal values are $P_a\text{co}_2$ 40 mmHg, $\dot{V}\text{co}_2$ 200 ml/min and $\dot{V}_A$ about 4 l/min. The constant value of 0.863 is derived from combining various converting factors for gas volumes (STPD or BTPS), for millilitres to litres and for gas concentration to tension.

The alveolar or arterial carbon dioxide tension is thus inversely proportional to the alveolar ventilation. The alveolar or effective ventilation is the total ventilation minus the wasted ventilation (see Chapter 2).

Since the physiological dead-space includes any alveolar dead-space as well as the anatomical dead-space, and since alveolar dead-space is due to ventilation/blood flow inequality (specifically the presence of areas of increased V/Q ratio), it follows that abnormalities of lung function should be reflected in the measurement of arterial carbon dioxide tension (Fig. 6.1). However, the arterial carbon dioxide tension does not usually rise in such circumstances, because the central chemoreceptors respond by increasing ventilatory drive. The end result, instead, is a normal arterial carbon dioxide tension but at the expense of an increased total ventilation.

Hypercapnia may be due either to absolute hypoventilation or to failure to increase ventilation sufficiently in the face of an increased carbon dioxide production or increased dead-space (relative hypoventilation). The former type of hypoventilation may be referred to as ventilatory failure. Thus, although the alveolar or arterial carbon dioxide tension is indeed inversely proportional to alveolar ventilation, hypercapnia should not be equated with hypoventilation without additional qualification (see Chapter 7).

Arterial pH

The arterial pH gives the single most important item of information concerning the acid–base state of the body as a whole. Venous blood pH indicates the acid–base state only of those individual areas drained by the blood at the site of sampling. Mixed venous (pulmonary arterial) blood pH, of course, gives the same information on the overall acid–base state of the body as does arterial blood pH, but it is much less convenient to sample.

In acidosis or alkalosis the arterial pH is decreased or increased respectively. Strictly speaking, changes in arterial pH indicate acidaemia or alkalaemia, and the terms acidosis or alkalosis refer to those processes producing or tending to produce these changes.

The tiny concentration of hydrogen ions in the blood may be expressed in nmol/l (SI units) as well as in the traditional pH notation. Thus, a normal arterial pH of 7.40 corresponds to a hydrogen ion concentration of 40 nmol/l. Because pH is a logarithmic scale, quite large changes in hydrogen ion concentration seem small when expressed as pH. For example, doubling or halving the hydrogen ion concentration to 80 or 20 nmol/l corresponds to a pH of 7.10 or 7.70 respectively. In fact, the pH may be the more 'physiological' notation, in that the consequences of change in hydrogen ion concentration tend to be proportionate to the log of its activity.

The relationship between any acid, its base and the hydrogen ion concentration is given as:

$$HB \rightleftharpoons B^- \times H^+$$

Since the major acid−base system in the body derives from carbon dioxide, namely carbonic acid/bicarbonate, this relationship is given as:

$$H_2CO_3 \rightleftharpoons HCO_3^- \times H^+$$

From this, Henderson's equation is derived:

$$(H^+) \propto \frac{(H_2CO_3)}{(HCO_3^-)} = 24 \frac{Pco_2}{(HCO_3^-)}$$

The concentration of carbonic acid or (H_2CO_3) is directly proportional to the Pco_2. The constant value of 24 (or 25) is derived from combining the dissociation constant and the solubility of carbon dioxide in plasma for a given pressure, and allowing for the conversion of mmol to nmol. The normal values for Henderson's equation are:

$$40 \text{ nmol/l} = 24 \frac{40 \text{ mmHg}}{24 \text{ mmol/l}}$$

This relationship in pH notation is the Henderson−Hasselbalch equation:

$$pH = pKa + \log \frac{HCO_3^-}{0.03 \, Pco_2}$$

Again, the normal values are:

$$7.4 = 6.1 + \log \frac{24}{0.03 \times 40}$$
$$= 6.1 + \log 20$$
$$= 6.1 + 1.3$$

Both the Henderson and Henderson−Hasselbalch equations enable calculation of the third variable, given the value of any two. In practice, the pH and Pco_2 are measured and the HCO_3^- calculated, usually from a programme within the analyser itself.

The Henderson–Hasselbalch equation has been paraphrased as:

$$pH = pKa + \log \frac{kidneys}{lungs}$$

At once, it can be seen that there must he only two forms of acidosis or alkalosis, namely respiratory or metabolic ('renal').

The four primary acid–base disturbances are shown in Table 6.1 in the form in which they originally occur. However, since the hydrogen ion concentration is usually kept within narrow limits by powerful homeostatic mechanisms, the end-result is a state at least partially compensated, as shown in Table 6.2. Clearly, respiratory mechanisms must compensate for metabolic disturbances and vice versa.

Table 6.1. The four primary acid–base disturbances

	Acidosis		Alkalosis	
	Respiratory	Metabolic	Respiratory	Metabolic
pH	↓	↓	↑	↑
P_aCO_2	↑	N	↓	N
HCO_3^-	N	↓	N	↑

Table 6.2. Compensated acid–base disturbances

	Acidosis				Alkalosis			
	Respiratory		Metabolic		Respiratory		Metabolic	
pH	↓	(N)	↓	(N)	↑	(N)	↑	(N)
P_aCO_2	↑*	↑*	N	↓†	↓*	↓*	N	(↑)†
HCO_3^-	N	↑†	↓*	↓*	N	↓†	↑*	↑*

* Primary, underlying change. † Secondary, compensatory response.

The causes of respiratory acidosis are alveolar hypoventilation, either total or relative (see Chapter 7). The causes of respiratory alkalosis are pulmonary parenchymal disease (with or without hypoxaemia), pulmonary vascular disease, central nervous system disease (especially mid-brain lesions), and a variety of systemic disorders such as fever, septicaemia, liver disease and salicylate intoxication; sometimes it is anxiety-related.

Metabolic compensation for respiratory acid–base disorders comes initially from a small, rapid change in bicarbonate from blood buffers and later from a larger, delayed change of renal origin. The latter response comprises a 2–4 mmol/l increase and a 3–6 mmol/l decrease in bicarbonate for a 10 mmHg increase or decrease respectively in carbon dioxide tension.

Respiratory compensation for metabolic acid−base disorders is rapid in onset but may have a lag in offset because of the blood−brain barrier to bicarbonate. The response comprises a 1−1.5 mmHg decrease and a 0.5−0.7 mmHg increase in carbon dioxide tension for a 1 mmol/l decrease or increase respectively in bicarbonate.

The total profile of an acid−base state is thus given by the pH, Pco_2 and HCO_3^-. If the pH is abnormal, the cause can be sought from the other two variables. In the compensated state, it can be difficult to decide which is the abnormal mechanism and which is the compensatory one. For example, respiratory acidosis and metabolic alkalosis compensate for each other, and it can be difficult to determine which came first in an individual patient. The solution to this problem is firstly, that compensation is rarely perfect and does not over-shoot, and thus that the residual direction of pH abnormality is likely to be the original, and secondly, that other clinical information is usually important, such as known lung disease, metabolic disorder (e.g. diabetes) or drug therapy.

Finally, mixed primary acid−base disturbances are also common. These are most frequently combined respiratory acidosis and metabolic alkalosis, and combined respiratory and metabolic acidosis. The former is seen in patients with chronic lung disease on treatment with corticosteroids and diuretics and the latter in patients with combined respiratory and renal failure or, in its most extreme form, in cardiac arrest. Combined respiratory and metabolic acidosis is clearly a dangerous situation, since no compensatory mechanism remains available.

7 Respiratory Failure

Definition

Respiratory failure is defined as the presence of hypoxaemia and/or hypercapnia, due to respiratory disease, at rest and at sea level. The degrees of hypoxaemia and hypercapnia chosen for this definition are usually P_aO_2 below 60 mmHg and P_aCO_2 above 50 mmHg, respectively.

The inclusion of hypoxaemia and hypercapnia in the definition of respiratory failure is expected, since oxygen and carbon dioxide exchange is the prime function of the lungs. What makes respiratory failure different from other organ dysfunction is the numerical precision with which it may be defined. However, this precision should not obscure the somewhat arbitrary nature of the levels of P_aO_2 and P_aCO_2 chosen.

Although hypoxaemia and hypercapnia commonly occur together, they frequently occur independently of each other, which is not surprising since their mechanisms are to a large extent different. Hypoxaemia without hypercapnia is seen in conditions of pulmonary disease with well preserved and sometimes increased respiratory drive (indeed, hypocapnia is commonly found). Hypercapnia without hypoxaemia is seen in conditions of depressed respiratory drive with normal lungs (although hypoxaemia must occur if the hypoventilation is sufficiently marked). These two types of respiratory failure are sometimes referred to as 'gas exchange failure' (or 'alveolar-capillary failure') and 'ventilatory failure'.

The caveat that respiratory failure must be due to respiratory disease may seem at first sight unnecessary, until it is remembered that right-to-left intracardiac shunting is also a cause of hypoxaemia.

Time-course

Respiratory failure may be acute, chronic or acute-on-chronic. The term acute implies a time-course of minutes to hours (or perhaps, at the most, days), there may or may not be previous underlying respiratory disease and there is little or no compensation. The term chronic implies a time-course of weeks to months (or perhaps even longer), the presence usually of significant underlying respiratory disease and evidence of compensation. The term acute-on-chronic does not imply a separate time-course but indicates that an acute exacerbation has occurred in the setting of long-standing failure.

The importance of making these distinctions is to guide decisions concerning both the speed and the goals of treatment.

Causes

The causes of respiratory failure are many and have been classified in various ways. One practical way is shown in Table 7.1. The common clinical settings in which respiratory failure occurs are shown in Table 7.2.

Table 7.1. Causes of respiratory failure

Gas exchange (alveolar-capillary) failure
hypoxaemia without hypercapnia:
- airways disease:
    asthma, chronic bronchitis, emphysema
- parenchymal disease:
    pneumonia, interstitial disease, oedema
- vascular disease:
    thromboembolism, vasculitis

Ventilatory failure
hypercapnia usually with hypoxaemia:
- mechanical load abnormalities:
    severe obstruction
- chest wall and respiratory muscle abnormalities:
    trauma, kyphoscoliosis, myasthenia
- central drive abnormalities:
    drugs, neurological disease

Table 7.2. Clinical settings of respiratory failure

Pulmonary disease
    chronic airways obstruction
    interstitial disease
    infection
    other insults (aspiration, near-drowning, toxic inhalation)
Other organ failure
    acute left heart failure
    cardiac arrest
    renal failure
Postoperative
Trauma
    pulmonary damage
    pneumothorax/haemothorax
    chest wall injury
Adult respiratory distress syndrome
Poisoning
Neuromuscular
    central
    peripheral

Clinical features

Hypoxaemia

The clinical manifestations of hypoxaemia are chiefly neurological, but also include circulatory changes, respiratory effects and cyanosis. However, all the clinical features of hypoxaemia are non-specific. While important, they can do no more than

67/*Respiratory Failure*

raise the suspicion of hypoxaemia. Its presence and degree can be assessed only by direct measurement.

• The dominance of the *neurological features* is not surprising in view of the brain's requirement for continuous oxygenation, manifest for example by unconsciousness within 10 sec if the circulation stops. The neurological changes are those of acute delirium. They include:

1 Impairment of highest functions, with headache, dizziness, restlessness, fatigue and insomnia (at mild levels of hypoxaemia).

2 Behavioural changes, weakness and decreased sensation to stimuli including pain (at moderate levels of hypoxaemia).

3 Unconsciousness, convulsions and death (at severe levels of hypoxaemia).

The neurological effects of hypoxaemia are thus those of central nervous system depression and have been justly compared with those of intoxication.

• The *circulatory features* are tachycardia with increased cardiac output, a generally unchanged blood pressure, increased pulmonary vascular resistance and pulmonary artery pressure, and redistribution of regional blood flow to increase coronary, cerebral and possibly renal blood flow. These circulatory features are modified by age, disease, drugs and anaesthesia. In particular, the heart rate response to hypoxaemia is reduced with age, is abolished by atropine and beta-blocking drugs, and is reversed with controlled ventilation.

• The *respiratory effects* are increased tidal volume and especially respiratory rate and thus total ventilation, increased airway resistance and thus work of breathing, and dyspnoea. The respiratory effects of hypoxaemia, and in particular the ventilatory responses, are blunted by age, obesity, sedative drugs, dopamine, airways obstruction, bilateral carotid surgery, dysautonomia, and sometimes on an idiopathic or even a familial basis.

• *Cyanosis* is popularly conceived as an important feature of hypoxaemia but, in fact, it is a late and unreliable sign. Central cyanosis is said to require the presence of about 5 g/dl of reduced haemoglobin. Thus, if the haemoglobin concentration is normal, the arterial saturation would need to be less than 75% (equivalent to a P_aO_2 of 40 mmHg) before cyanosis could be detected with certainty. In practice, these traditionally quoted values are considerable overestimates of the degree of hypoxaemia required, since cyanosis can usually be detected at much higher levels of arterial saturation (e.g. 85% or more). In general, cyanosis is detectable earlier in polycythaemia or with experience and later in anaemia, if there is dark skin pigmentation or with poor lighting. Central and peripheral cyanosis are not always easily separable and may coexist.

While the effects of hypoxaemia are assessed clinically and the degree measured directly, it is also instructive to assess hypoxaemia in relation to altitude. An example is shown in Table 7.3.

Table 7.3. Altitude and quantification of hypoxia

Altitude (m/ft)	Barometric pressure (mmHg)	P_IO_2 (mmHg)	P_aO_2 (mmHg)	S_aO_2 (%)	Symptoms, if healthy
Sea level	760	150	100	97	Nil
2500/8000	560	110	60	90	Exertional impairment
3500/12 000	480	90	50	85	Headache, breathlessness on exertion
5500/18 000	380	70	40	75	Severe breathlessness, pulmonary oedema, mental impairment
9000/30 000	230	40	20	30	Death

Values are approximate and are for breathing air. 18 000 feet is the highest level at which permanent human habitation is possible but much higher levels (29 000 ft) have been reached by acclimatized and specially trained climbers without using oxygen.

Hypoxaemia sufficiently severe to cause tissue hypoxia may be quantified by measuring markers of anaerobic tissue metabolism. Such hypoxia occurs when oxygen delivery is less than oxygen requirements, resulting in oxygen debt. This is manifest by increased blood lactate and decreased pH, and invariably occurs if the P_aO_2 is in the region of 30 mmHg.

Hypoxaemia (decreased arterial oxygen tension) is, of course, only one of the causes of hypoxia (decreased tissue oxygenation). As shown in Table 7.4, hypoxia may be due to circulatory (cardiac output), haematological (haemoglobin) and peripheral abnormalities as well as to respiratory failure. In turn, hypoxaemia may be caused by a number of mechanisms (Table 7.5), of which ventilation/blood flow inequality is the most common.

Table 7.4. Causes of hypoxia

Traditional nomenclature	Current nomenclature
(Barcroft, 1920)	
Anoxic	Arterial hypoxaemia
Anaemic	Abnormal O_2 carriage
Stagnant	Abnormal O_2 delivery
(Peters and Van Slyke, 1931)	
Histotoxic	Mitochondrial disease

Table 7.5. Causes of hypoxaemia

Causes	A-a Po_2 gradient
Reduced inspired oxygen tension Alveolar hypoventilation	Normal
Ventilation/blood flow mismatching Veno-arterial shunting Impaired diffusion	Increased

69/*Respiratory Failure*

The clinical manifestations of hypercapnia are chiefly circulatory and neurological but also include respiratory effects. Their expression seems related more to the rate of development of hypercapnia than to its severity. As with hypoxaemia, all the clinical features of hypercapnia are non-specific. They are, however, characteristic and in the appropriate context should raise the suspicion of hypercapnia. Again, as with hypoxaemia, the presence and degree of hypercapnia can be assessed only by direct measurement.

• The *circulatory features* are vasodilatation, increased arterial systolic and pulse pressure, bounding pulse, tachycardia and sweating. The circulatory changes are thus those of the acute hyperdynamic state, with many similarities to those seen in fever, anaemia or thyrotoxicosis.

• The *neurological features* are those of confusion, drowsiness, even narcosis and coma. There may be apathy, loss of concentration, irritability, headache and anorexia. Examination may show twitching, decreased tendon reflexes, upgoing plantar reflexes, pupillary constriction and retinal venous engorgement. The neurological changes are thus reminiscent of the narcosis produced by opiates.

• The *respiratory features* may include dyspnoea if the hypercapnia is acute. If there is absolute hypoventilation, a reduced tidal volume and/or respiratory rate may be clinically evident.

Mechanical changes

Mechanical abnormalities of the lungs and/or chest wall are frequently present in patients with respiratory failure. In general, it is the presence of a significant mechanical abnormality rather than hypoxaemia or hypercapnia that is responsible for the specific respiratory symptom of dyspnoea in patients with respiratory failure.

• *Airflow limitation* is the commonest result of mechanical changes. In airways obstruction, it is particularly noted in expiration and is usually associated with audible wheeze or with rhonchi on auscultation. There is a prolonged expiratory time and the patient may have difficulty speaking without being continually interrupted by the need to take the next breath. Airflow limitation may also occur in interstitial lung disease. It is then noted particularly during inspiration, which is cut short prematurely. A shortening of the inspiratory time to less than 1 sec is a useful bedside indication of increased ventilatory work in such situations.

• *Hyperinflation* of the chest is seen in patients with long-standing airways obstruction. Other mechanical abnormalities of the chest wall which may be associated with respiratory failure include acute changes, such as following trauma, and chronic changes, such as in kyphoscoliosis.

Other features

As with any organ failure, respiratory failure may be associated with features indicative of underlying disease, precipitating factors, compensatory mechanisms and complications.

• *Underlying disease* may be present in acute respiratory

failure and is inevitable in chronic respiratory failure. Airways obstruction, such as in asthma, chronic bronchitis or emphysema, is the most common feature but virtually any disorder of the lungs or chest wall may at times be found.

• *Precipitating factors* are of importance in tipping the balance in patients with established respiratory disease but not currently in failure. The most important precipitating factors are infections and drugs. Chest infection is a common cause of acute exacerbation of chronic lung disease. Any sedative drugs, but particularly narcotics, have the potential to precipitate respiratory failure in patients with precarious respiratory drive. Uncontrolled oxygen therapy has a similar effect by eliminating the hypoxic ventilatory drive in patients whose normal carbon dioxide drive has been lost, usually as a result of chronic hypercapnia. Needless to say, acute withdrawal of bronchodilator agents or corticosteroids may also precipitate respiratory failure in susceptible patients.

• *Compensatory mechanisms* may be clinically evident, particularly tachycardia, hyperventilation, polycythaemia in hypoxaemia and hyperinflation in airways obstruction. The presence of polycythaemia implies that hypoxaemia must have been both considerable (P_aO_2 less than 60 mmHg) and persistent (at least weeks).

• *Complications* include, most importantly, other organ failure in response to respiratory failure. The chief complication is *cor pulmonale* or right heart failure, particularly when hypercapnia has been prominent or when pulmonary vascular obliteration is a feature of the underlying respiratory disease.

Assessment

Clinical

The clinical assessment of patients with respiratory failure is uniquely able to establish the time-course of the process, the patient's previous health and thus the current therapeutic goal, and the patient's tolerance of the level of disability. The history and examination also indicate much about the patient's responses to hypoxaemia and hypercapnia, and the presence of mechanical abnormalities, underlying disease, precipitating factors, compensatory mechanisms and complications.

Arterial blood gas analysis

Arterial blood gas analysis is required to confirm the diagnosis of respiratory failure and its type, to quantify it and to follow its progress. As previously indicated, hypoxaemia and hypercapnia can be documented only by direct measurement.

Of particular practical importance is the response of the arterial oxygen and carbon dioxide tensions to oxygen administration. If the arterial oxygen tension fails to increase, or if a modest increase is accompanied by a significant increase in arterial carbon dioxide tension, the need for mechanical ventilation becomes more likely.

If hypercapnia is present, its chronicity can be assessed from the blood bicarbonate concentration. Renal compensation for an increased arterial carbon dioxide tension is by retention of bicarbonate, a mechanism which takes a few days to become fully operative. Thus, for example, an elevated arterial carbon dioxide tension with an appropriately decreased pH and normal bicarbonate concentration implies that the hypercapnia is very recent (and also much less likely to be aggravated by oxygen administration). On the other hand, an elevated arterial carbon dioxide tension with a normal pH and therefore concomitantly increased bicarbonate concentration implies a more chronic process (and one that should not be reversed rapidly and completely).

Although respiratory acidosis is the expected finding in respiratory failure, primary metabolic alkalosis is also common in those patients who have been treated with corticosteroids and diuretics, and thus may be hypokalaemic, hypochloraemic and even hyponatraemic or hypovolaemic.

Chest X-ray

The chest X-ray examination is essential in all cases of respiratory failure to help clarify the cause, to exclude an acutely treatable problem, such as pneumothorax, and to confirm the correct positioning of any tubes and lines, such as an endotracheal tube or central venous catheter.

Laboratory investigations

• *Lung function tests* other than blood gas analysis are not usually practicable in patients with acute respiratory failure. In chronic respiratory failure, spirometry should always be performed together with such further tests as may be indicated by the nature of the particular underlying disease. Usually, these laboratory-based lung function tests are most informative when performed with the patient in a stable, 'at best' situation, since they may then help set future therapeutic goals.

• *Microbiological examination* of sputum is essential to confirm the presence and characterize the nature of suspected chest infection. *Haematological investigation* is required to demonstrate polycythaemia and *biochemical examination* to show any electrolyte abnormalities.

Table 7.6. Emergency measures for acute respiratory failure

Patent airway
 tongue, foreign body, intubation, tracheostomy
Pulmonary ventilation
 expired air, hand or mechanical ventilation
Oxygen enrichment
 if available
Circulatory resuscitation
 if cardiac arrest, full CPR
Bronchodilators
 if acute asthma
Expert assistance, transport

Management

Acute respiratory failure presenting as a medical emergency demands a patent airway and the movement of ventilating air. Expired air resuscitation after clearing the airways can be life-saving in situations such as electrocution, envenomation, cardiac arrest, and pharyngeal or laryngeal obstruction. The emergency measures for these acute situations are summarized in Table 7.6.

The general principles of the management of respiratory failure are listed in Table 7.7. The individual therapeutic modalities are considered in greater detail in Chapter 8 (Respiratory Therapy).

Table 7.7. General principles of management of respiratory failure

Oxygen
Bronchodilators
Humidification
Removal of tracheobronchial secretions
Artificial airway
Mechanical ventilation (IPPV)
Positive end-expiratory pressure (PEEP) or continuous positive
    airway pressure (CPAP)
Antibiotics
Other drugs:
    respiratory stimulants
    mucolytic agents
    expectorants

Respiratory Therapy

Oxygen
Bronchodilators
Humidification and aerosol therapy
Removal of tracheobronchial
  secretions
Artificial airway
Mechanical ventilation

Positive end-expiratory pressure
  (PEEP) and continuous
  positive airway pressure
  (CPAP)
Antibiotics
Other drugs

Oxygen

Oxygen is best considered as a potent drug. It has indications, contraindications, dosage and side-effects.

● The *indication* for oxygen is hypoxaemia from any cause. However, right-to-left shunting responds little to increased inspired oxygen and pure ventilatory failure requires additionally the restoration of ventilation. The most common cause of hypoxaemia is ventilation/blood flow inequality, particularly the presence of low ventilation/blood flow ratios (see Chapter 2). Oxygen may be of minor benefit in non-hypoxaemic causes of hypoxia by increasing the arterial oxygen content somewhat, due to slightly higher oxygen saturation and slightly more dissolved oxygen. Hypoxaemia is best formally documented by arterial blood gas analysis. However, it may be inferred if there are appropriate clinical features or in known situations (e.g. acute pulmonary oedema).

● There are no absolute *contraindications* to oxygen therapy, provided there is a clear indication. Caution should be exercised and the lowest effective dose used, particularly in chronic respiratory failure with hypercapnia, in premature infants, and in patients who have previously received bleomycin, since this latter agent seems to predispose more readily to serious oxygen toxicity.

● The *dose* of oxygen should be the minimum required to relieve the symptoms of hypoxia and to normalize the arterial oxygen tension. The duration of oxygen therapy should be that required for the original indication to resolve.

● The *side-effects* of oxygen are:

(a) Respiratory depression in patients with chronic hypercapnia who had been relying on hypoxaemia for respiratory drive (relief of hypoxia must still take precedence, even if the consequence is exacerbation of hypercapnia requiring mechanical ventilation).

(b) Pulmonary oxygen toxicity (bronchopulmonary dysplasia) after prolonged administration.

(c) Retrolental fibroplasia in premature infants.

In practice, oxygen may be given by a variety of devices. Nasal cannulae (prongs) with oxygen flow at 2–4 l/min are the most comfortable, practical and inexpensive method for general use when the desired inspired oxygen concentration is approximately 25—35%. A nasal catheter can also be used. Simple face-masks with oxygen flow at 4—10 l/min or more are relatively comfortable and most effective for general use when the desired inspired oxygen concentration is approximately 25—50%. Venturi face-masks are used when an exact inspired oxygen concentration is required, e.g. 24%, 28%, 35%. Reservoir face-masks are used when higher inspired oxygen concentration levels are required, e.g. 60% or more. It is hard to achieve much higher inspired oxygen concentrations with a face-mask unless it is close-fitting and of the anaesthetic type, when up to 100% may be obtained. A face trough may be used when a face-mask is not tolerated and only modest inspired oxygen concentrations are required. Patients with a tracheostomy may receive oxygen via a tracheostomy mask or a T-piece. Oxygen tents are no longer used in adults as they are cumbersome and expensive. The use of a ventilator with an oxygen blender permits exact control of the inspired oxygen concentration at any level between 21 and 100%. As a rough guide, if an inspired oxygen concentration of greater than 40% is required to correct hypoxaemia, mechanical ventilation or continuous positive airway pressure will commonly be needed.

Inspired oxygen concentrations of up to 40% can apparently be tolerated for long periods without producing significant oxygen toxicity. About this concentration and certainly above 60%, bronchopulmonary dysplasia becomes increasingly evident with time, although its occurrence is not inevitable. These changes are probably dose—time dependent.

Bronchodilators

Bronchodilators are indicated in patients with generalized airways obstructions, even if not overtly asthmatic. They may also be helpful in other patients since they enhance mucociliary clearance. Bronchodilators are best given as β_2 sympathomimetic agonists by nebulizer and as aminophylline and corticosteroids by intravenous infusion. The use of bronchodilators is discussed in greater detail in Chapter 10 (Asthma).

Humidification and aerosol therapy

Humidification of the inspired air is required if the tracheobronchial secretions are viscid or inspissated, or if an artificial airway is being used for more than a brief period. Humidification is achieved by passing the inspired gas through a heated, water-filled device. To prevent later rain-out, a heated delivery hose may be used. With heated devices, the temperature of the inspired gas of the patient should be monitored and in more sophisticated designs this temperature may servocontrol the water temperature in the humidifier chamber. The most effective humidification is achieved when the device is part of a ventilator circuit and is connected to the patient via an endotracheal or tracheostomy tube. Heated humidifiers are complex and expensive, both to buy and to maintain, although relatively simple disposable systems have recently become available. Non-heated humidifiers are relatively ineffective.

Nebulizers may also be used to deliver water to the tracheo-bronchial tree. Unlike humidifiers, which deliver water vapour, nebulizers deliver water particles. They are thus more readily a source of bacterial contamination. An ultrasonic nebulizer delivers very large amounts of particulate water in a short time and may sometimes be used in selected patients. Nowadays, nebulizers are used mostly for intermittent, inhaled drug administration (aerosol therapy) rather than for continuous water delivery.

The simplest nebulizers are the popular metered aerosols which are inhaled through the mouth. Aerosols may also be generated by compressed gas or a pump using a venturi-operated nebulizer chamber and a face-mask. Many believe this to be more effective, though less simple, than a metered aerosol device. Aerosols may easily be administered to intubated and mechanically ventilated patients by similar nebulizers sited in the inspiratory circuit. Particulate water is a bronchoconstrictor and should be avoided, especially in asthmatics for whom bronchodilator solutions should always be diluted in saline before nebulization.

Removal of tracheobronchial secretions

Tracheobronchial secretions need to be cleared in all patients. Additional requirements occur in those either with excessive secretions or unable to clear their own secretions. Physiotherapy (physical therapy) is directed towards helping patients clear their own secretions by posturing, percussion and vibration, and by deep breathing and coughing.

In intubated patients, direct tracheobronchial suctioning with a sterile catheter may be performed. It is frequently combined with physiotherapy. This important manoeuvre must be carried out in a strictly aseptic manner, so that it does not introduce micro-organisms into the unprotected respiratory tract. Suction catheters reach as far as the carina and right main bronchus; coudé-tipped catheters can be used to enter the left main bronchus. A catheter can often be passed via the nose through the vocal cords and into the upper trachea in non-intubated patients but this is not always an easy technique.

Difficult secretions may also be removed during fibreoptic bronchoscopy, even in intubated patients. This technique also permits lavage and repeated suctioning under vision until an obstructed area is cleared. Tracheobronchial secretions obtained with a sterile catheter or a bronchoscope are valuable specimens for microbiological examination.

Artificial airway

Endotracheal intubation is the most readily available means of providing a reliable artifical airway. An endotracheal tube provides airway patency via its central lumen and airway protection by an inflatable cuff. Measures less complex (position, oropharyngeal or nasopharyngeal airway) or more complex (tracheostomy) are also often employed. The general indications for endotracheal intubation are shown in Table 8.1.

Airway patency and protection is a major priority in all

Table 8.1. Indications for endotracheal intubation

Airway patency and protection
Tracheobronchial toilet
Connection to ventilator

patients unable to protect their own airway, i.e. with impaired conscious state or reduced cough and gag reflexes. If the patient's disability in this regard is both incomplete and temporary, it is often satisfactory to put the patient in the postanaesthetic position (semi-prone, slightly head down), preferably with an oropharyngeal airway.

Access for repeated tracheobronchial toilet is required if physiotheraphy alone is insufficient and a single fibreoptic bronchoscopy is inappropriate. Long-term partial access in poorly cooperative patients may also be obtained with a nasopharyngeal airway through which a suction catheter can be passed.

It is difficult to connect the various means of positive pressure support to a patient without a cuffed endotracheal or tracheostomy tube. However, for short-term use in cooperative patients, a close-fitting anaesthetic type mask may sometimes be successfully employed, either for mechanical ventilation or more commonly for continuous positive airway pressure.

An endotracheal tube may be passed either orally or nasally. An oral tube is easier to insert (or replace) and can usually have a large lumen. A nasal tube is more stable and usually more comfortable. Modern tubes are of smooth plastic and have high-volume, low-pressure cuffs to minimize airway damage. Such tubes may be left in place for at least a week and often much longer.

The indications for tracheostomy are listed in Table 8.2. While most of these are elective, some clearly occur in emergency situations. In these situations, cricothyroid puncture may be more appropriate than formal tracheostomy.

Table 8.2. Indications for tracheostomy

Prolonged intubation
1 week, possibly much longer
Upper airway damage
e.g. trauma, burns, postintubation
Difficult intubation
e.g. fractured jaw and great difficulty anticipated in the event of re-intubation
Surgery
e.g. laryngectomy
Ease and safety of nursing care
especially if facilities limited
Patient tolerance
but try nasotracheal tube first
Reduce dead-space
rare

Mechanical ventilation

The indications for use of a ventilator are listed in Table 8.3. The first two indications are by far the most important.

● *Inadequate ventilation* is the classical indication for mechanical ventilation. This type of respiratory failure may be referred to as 'ventilatory failure'. The patient's ventilation is inadequate to meet the metabolic needs and, as previously discussed when considering the arterial carbon dioxide tension, there may or may not be absolute hypoventilation. Patients with inadequate ventilation have been described as those who either 'won't breathe' (i.e. a central mechanism with resultant impaired effort) or 'can't breathe' (i.e. a peripheral mechanism associated with too much respiratory work and often coincidentally with abnormal gas exchange).

Table 8.3. Indications for mechanical ventilation

Inadequate ventilation
Hypoxaemia
Flail chest
Acute pulmonary oedema
Physiotherapy?

The diagnosis of inadequate ventilation is suspected on clinical examination, supported by measurement of tidal volume, respiratory rate and minute ventilation, and confirmed by measurement of arterial carbon dioxide tension. Initial therapeutic measures should ensure care with sedative drugs or excessive oxygen. Analeptic drugs may occasionally be useful, for example naloxone in narcotic overdose.

● *Hypoxaemia* is a less obvious indication for mechanical ventilation. This type of respiratory failure is not usually associated with hypercapnia and may be referred to as 'gas exchange failure' or 'alveolar-capillary failure'. It has been appreciated as a legitimate indication for mechanical ventilation only in relatively recent times. If hypoxaemia is clinically significant and has failed to respond to oxygen administration, and attention has been paid to any immediately reversible conditions (e.g. pneumothorax, asthma), then mechanical ventilation should be considered. This will generally result in an increased arterial oxygen tension, even for the same inspired oxygen concentration and same alveolar ventilation. This improvement results perhaps because mechanical ventilation gives a better ventilatory pattern and distribution of ventilation, perhaps because there is less respiratory work and oxygen consumption, but most likely because intermittent positive pressure ventilation may reverse alveolar closure and airway collapse. Positive end-expiratory pressure or continuous positive airway pressure is an extension of this mechanism of action and the adult respiratory distress syndrome is the best clinical example for this application. Mechanical ventilation does not improve oxygenation in normal lungs. A general rule is that mechanical ventilation is indicated for hypoxaemia if the arterial oxygen tension is less than 60 mmHg despite an inspired oxygen concentration of 40% or more, or if the patient is exhausted.

- *Flail chest*, if severe, is a strong indication for mechanical ventilation (see Chapter 14). This should be considered if there is significant gas exchange impairment though, as subsequently discussed, this is usually due more to underlying pulmonary contusion than to the consequences of the chest wall damage itself. Mechanical ventilation may also be required if the patient is exhausted or uncooperative, or occasionally if the chest wall damage is so severe that healing and moulding will be impaired resulting in significant chest wall deformity.

- *Acute pulmonary oedema*, if fulminating and unresponsive to usual medical measures, generally responds rapidly and often dramatically to mechanical ventilation.

- *Physiotherapy* should not nowadays be regarded as a legitimate indication in most patients for the use of a ventilator. It is generally inappropriate to use such expensive machines for such simple tasks. However, there probably remains a place for the use of a ventilator in selected patients who are unable to take a sufficiently large breath for themselves despite encouragement and incentive breathing devices.

The ventilator should always be set such that the combination of pressure, flow and time gives not only appropriate total ventilation but also optimal distribution of ventilation within the lungs. The usual goal is to achieve normal arterial blood gas values, though compromises may be accepted in special circumstances. A second goal is to render 'respiratory satisfaction' by ensuring that the ventilator and the patient are well matched so as to provide patient comfort with minimal sedation.

Modern ventilators all operate by applying intermittent positive pressure to the airway. This mode of ventilation is called intermittent positive pressure ventilation (IPPV). Traditionally, mechanical ventilation has been in either the control mode (CMV) or assist mode (Fig. 8.1). In the former, the machine has completely taken over the rhythm of ventilation. In the latter, the patient may initiate inspiration, i.e. assist or trigger the ventilator, which then delivers the set tidal volume.

Recently, other ventilatory modes have been introduced. *Intermittent mandatory ventilation* (IMV) is a form of partial ventilatory support where a certain number of mandatory breaths come from the machine and the rest can be taken by the patient unaided (Fig. 8.1). IMV was introduced as a means of weaning patients from prolonged periods of mechanical ventilation, but more recently it has become popular as a primary means of ventilatory support. Its purported advantages in this setting are less average airway pressure, less barotrauma, less circulatory depression, less hyperventilation and less sedation. It is usually combined with CPAP.

High-frequency ventilation (HFV) is an interesting new modality achieved either by positive pressure ventilation, jet

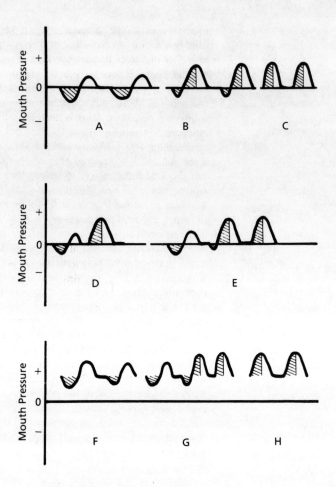

Fig. 8.1. Various types of positive pressure ventilation techniques illustrated by the cycle of airway pressure. Hatched areas represent inspiration and clear areas expiration. (A) Spontaneous breathing. (B) Intermittent positive pressure ventilation (IPPV) (assist mode). (C) Intermittent positive pressure ventilation (IPPV) (control mode). (D) Intermittent mandatory ventilation (IMV). (E) Synchronized intermittent mandatory ventilation (SIMV). (F) Spontaneous breathing plus CPAP. (G) SIMV plus CPAP. (H) IPPV (control mode) plus PEEP.

ventilation or oscillations. It appears to offer particular benefit in mechanically ventilated patients with bronchopleural fistula, barotrauma and in some infants. Its mechanisms and role are still uncertain and special machines are required.

Positive end-expiratory pressure (PEEP) and continuous positive airway pressure (CPAP)

Normally the end of expiration occurs when the pressure in the airway falls to zero (with respect to atmospheric pressure). This applies both during spontaneous breathing and mechanical ventilation. If the airway pressure during expiration is not allowed to fall to zero, i.e. remains positive, the patient has to breathe 'further up' his pressure−volume curve to achieve the same ventilation. Lung volumes, especially FRC, are increased. Areas of the lung which may have been below their closing volume during the latter part of expiration may now be kept open during the whole respiratory cycle. Ventilation/blood flow abnormalities contributing to venous admixture and right-to-left shunting may be improved and arterial oxygen tension increased. However, the effects of PEEP or CPAP on the circulation are depressant, with a tendency to increased cardiac filling pressures and reduced venous return and cardiac output. In using PEEP or CPAP, therefore, it is important to be sure that any respiratory advantages outweight any cardiovascular disadvantages.

PEEP refers to the manoeuvre which ensures that the airway pressure remains positive during expiration (Fig. 8.1). The term PEEP is usually used in relation to mechanical ventilation. CPAP refers to the manoeuvre which ensures that the airway pressure remains positive during the whole of the respiratory cycle (Fig. 8.1). The form of CPAP achieved when mechanical ventilation and PEEP are used is called continuous positive pressure ventilation (CPPV). PEEP and CPAP are virtually interchangeable terms.

● The *indication* for PEEP or CPAP is hypoxaemia. As a rough guide, PEEP or CPAP should be used if the arterial oxygen tension is less than 60 mmHg despite an inspired oxygen concentration of 60% or more (i.e. '60−60 rule') and provided acutely reversible factors have been excluded (e.g. pneumothorax, tube misplacement, sputum plugging, etc.). The best clinical example is the adult respiratory distress syndrome.

● The *contraindications* to PEEP or CPAP are all relative and are listed in Table 8.4.

● The *optimal level* of PEEP or CPAP is generally between 5−15 cmH$_2$O. The selection of the optimal level of PEEP or CPAP has been much argued and presently two views predominate. Firstly, PEEP or CPAP could be set so as to maximize oxygen transport, i.e. to take into account not only any beneficial effect on arterial oxygenation but also any deleterious effect on cardiac output. Secondly, PEEP or CPAP could be used for its oxygen-sparing effect, i.e. its level

Table 8.4. Contraindications to PEEP

Conditions	Comments
Chronic airways obstruction	FRC already high
Chronic restrictive lung disease	FRC irreversibly low
Pneumothorax	
Bronchopleural fistula	
Unilateral lung disease	Aggravated by PEEP
Circulatory impairment	
Neurological damage	PEEP harmful
Normal lung	Probably unjustified

could be adjusted so as to permit the inspired oxygen concentration to be able to be reduced to 60% or less. This latter view is probably the more attractive.

There are two important potential *complications* of PEEP or CPAP:

1 *Circulatory impairment* may occur in some patients with either cardiovascular dysfunction or hypovolaemia. This effect is variable and usually minor but should be monitored in appropriate patients with suitable haemodynamic measurements.

2 *Barotrauma*, especially pneumothorax, but also mediastinal emphysema, interstitial pulmonary emphysema and subcutaneous emphysema, is a potential complication of mechanical ventilation, especially if inspired pressures are high or PEEP is used. There is no direct correlation, however, between the occurrence of barotrauma and the level of pressure used.

Antibiotics

Antibiotics are obviously used in chest infections, the general principle being to use the antibiotic with the narrowest and most specific spectrum appropriate for the particular infection suspected or demonstrated. The initial antibiotic regimen may need modification when the microbiological results become available. Prophylactic antibiotics are generally contraindicated in chest disease. Penicillin or ampicillin (or amoxycillin) are the most generally useful antibiotics. Erythromycin is of value in atypical pneumonia or penicillin-sensitive patients. Aminoglycosides may be used in a number of Gram-negative infections and the third generation cephalosporins, or new broad-spectrum semi-synthetic penicillins, may also be of considerable value in these cases. Antibiotic therapy is discussed in greater detail in Chapter 12 (Respiratory Infections).

Other drugs

● *Respiratory stimulants* that could be of value in respiratory failure are not available, except for (a) naloxone in narcotic overdose, (b) possibly aminophylline to some degree (although its main use is as a bronchodilator) and (c) removal of respiratory depressant agents.

● *Mucolytic agents*, except for adequate humidification, are rarely indicated. Acetylcysteine is the best known such agent but is also a bronchial irritant.

● *Expectorants* are of no value in respiratory failure, since cough is usefully stimulated only by mechanical means.

9 Immunology and the Lung

Introduction

The lungs probably have a greater degree of contact with the environment than does any other organ. There is frequent and potentially massive exposure, not only to infecting organisms and allergens in the inspired air, but also to blood-borne organisms, toxic substances, immune complexes and activated cells from other sites in the body, as the whole of the venous return passes through the pulmonary capillary bed.

Immunity is one of the important mechanisms for the defence of the lungs against this variety of insults. The sterility of the alveolar environment is a reflection of the efficiency of these defences, whose elements, both specific and non-specific, local and systemic, interact as an integrated response.

Immune mechanisms

Immunological mechanisms in the lung operate at the mucosal surface and in the interstitium. These mechanisms act to remove antigen with minimal inflammatory response and thus minimal disturbance of lung function.

Specific immunity requires the cooperation of both humoral and cell-mediated mechanisms of defence. In particular, bronchial-associated lymphoid tissue, which forms part of the common mucosal immune system and contains both T and B cells, is responsible for antigen-specific immune responses.

IgA

This is secreted by plasma cells in the bronchial mucosa and is present in high concentration in the tracheobronchial secretions. It is the major immunoglobulin in the upper respiratory tract. IgA appears to protect the respiratory mucous membrane against the attachment of foreign particles, including organisms and proteins, and thus limits microbial expansion. Levels of secretory IgA correlate better with respiratory immunity to specific infections than do serum levels.

IgG

This is both produced locally and can be recruited from the systemic pool. It enhances phagocytosis by macrophages, particularly in the lower respiratory tract.

IgE

This is also secreted by plasma cells in the bronchial mucosa and, like IgA, is a mucosal antibody present in respiratory secretions. It is especially prominent in atopic individuals. IgE acts in association with local mast cells and enhances host defence by recruiting eosinophils, promoting smooth muscle contraction and mucus secretion, and increasing epithelial and endothelial permeability. IgE may thus function to protect the respiratory mucous membrane, perhaps against some parasites, but it is best known for its adverse effects as the reaginic antibody responsible for immediate (Type I) hypersensitivity reactions.

T lymphocytes

These are present in both the bronchial mucosa and the lumen. Some T lymphocytes are cytotoxic for antigen-bearing cells, such as those infected with viruses. Some modulate the immune response and thus inflammation. Some secrete lymphokines which, among other effects, activate macrophages, attract eosinophils and increase vascular permeability. T lymphocytes are responsible for delayed (Type IV) cell-mediated hypersensitivity reactions.

Complement

This is a series of plasma proteins that act as sequential enzymes. They are triggered by antigen−antibody reactions (classical pathway) or by endotoxin or bacterial cell walls (alternate pathway). Complement activation is typical of IgG reactions but does not occur in IgA or IgE responses. Complement activation results in phagocytosis and lysis of infecting organisms and other foreign cells, whether or not antibody has been involved. These effects are produced by opsonization, a coating which enhances phagocytosis. Some complement components have powerful additional effects in many aspects of the inflammatory response, e.g. in chemotaxis and vascular permeability.

Macrophages

These are normally present in the distal lumen of the lower respiratory tract, especially in the alveoli. Following activation, e.g. by lymphokines, they are responsible for ingesting and degrading a wide range of foreign particulate matter, as well as cellular debris, antigen and immune complexes. They are also important in processing antigen before its presentation to T cells.

Neutrophils

These are a key element in the acute inflammatory response following their mobilization by chemotactic factors. Many species of bacteria are readily phagocytosed by neutrophils, often after 'digestibility' has been improved by naturally-occurring opsonins. Neutrophils may also release a number of substances which have potent effects on adjacent cells.

Eosinophils

These contain enzymes which may inhibit histamine, leucotrienes and prostaglandins. They may play an important role in defence against parasites and are particularly associated with Type I hypersensitivity reactions. Charcot−Leyden crystals in the sputum of asthmatics are derived from degraded eosinophil cytoplasm.

Immunological abnormalities

Pulmonary disease may occur because of immunological deficiency or because of specific immunological reactions (hypersensitivity, autoimmunity).

Immunological deficiency

This occurs in a wide variety of forms. There may be congenital deficiency or abnormality of immunoglobulins, complement or cellular immunity. Acquired deficiencies include decreased antibody levels (hypogammaglobulinaemia, IgA deficiency, leukaemia, myeloma and other dysproteinaemias), decreased cell-mediated immunity (lymphoma, acquired immune deficiency syndrome), agranulocytosis, and non-specific interference by disease (diabetes, splenectomy) or therapy (corticosteroids, cytotoxic agents).

Immune deficiency predisposes to infection. An underlying immunodeficiency should always be sought in a patient with recurrent, severe or unusual chest infection. Deficient humoral immunity is associated particularly with pyogenic bacterial infections. Deficient cellular immunity is associated particularly with viral, fungal and pseudomonal infections. Both types of defective immunity can be associated with more exotic infections, e.g. due to *Pneumocystis carinii*.

Specific immunological reactions

These reactions, whereby antibody combines with antigen, can result in associated tissue damage as well as in destruction of the antigen. Responses causing tissue damage are called *hypersensitivity reactions* and are classified into four types.
• *Type I* (immediate, anaphylactic) is IgE-mediated, causing mast cell and basophil degranulation in the mucosa and lumen with liberation of mediators, e.g. histamine, leucotrienes, prostaglandins. The immediate airways obstruction in response to inhaled allergen may be followed after 4–8 hours by a late obstructive response, which is also usually IgE-mediated, probably with associated neutrophil or eosinophil involvement. Clinical pulmonary examples include allergic rhinitis and extrinsic asthma (both atopic diseases) and anaphylaxis.
• *Type II* (cytotoxic) is usually IgG-mediated, often with complement, and causes cell damage because antigen remains cell-bound. Clinical pulmonary examples include Goodpasture's syndrome, in which antibodies arise to the alveolar basement membrane.
• *Type III* (immune complex disease, Arthus reaction) involves the production of antigen–antibody complexes, usually with IgG and complement, and causes vascular damage, granulomas and eosinophilia. An important clinical example is the delayed-onset response to inhaled antigen which is seen in hypersensitivity pneumonitis (e.g. farmer's lung). Unlike the Type I response, it consists of restriction rather than obstruction and does not have an immediate component. Other clinical pulmonary examples include bronchopulmonary aspergillosis, asthmatic pulmonary eosinophilia, rheumatoid lung and possibly diffuse fibrosing alveolitis and a number of forms of

pulmonary vasculitis. These reactions tend not to be steroid-responsive (except for some early steps) but generally respond to cytotoxic agents.

● *Type IV* (cell-mediated, delayed) involves the reaction of antigen with sensitized T lymphocytes, causing release of lymphokines with mobilization of macrophages, local inflammation, vascular damage, granuloma formation and necrosis. A complex set of interactions occurs among the various subsets of lymphocytes to give rise to associated phenomena such as immune complex formation, auto-antibodies and cutaneous anergy. The release of interleukin 1 from activated macrophages probably mediates many systemic effects such as fever and weight loss. Clinical pulmonary examples include reactions to many viral, fungal and some bacterial diseases, graft rejection and some pulmonary granulomas. These reactions are generally steroid-responsive.

Auto-immune diseases include those with organ-specific antibodies (none are pulmonary) and those with antibodies which are non-organ-specific. The latter include the collagen-vascular (connective tissue) disorders which frequently involve the lung.

Pulmonary disease due to immune mechanisms

Many pulmonary diseases have well defined pathogenetic mechanisms of an immunological nature. Many others have a possible or probable immunological basis.

● *Pulmonary infections* may be associated with immune deficiency, as previously indicated above.

● *Allergic asthma and anaphylaxis* are usually associated with Type I hypersensitivity due to antigen-specific IgE on mast cells giving rise to mediator release. Direct mediator release not involving IgE may occur with or without complement involvement; examples include reactions to aspirin and radiographic contrast media and in these cases no previous contact is requried. Generalized degranulation of mast cells, which is IgE-mediated, is called anaphylaxis and similar reactions which are not IgE-mediated are called anaphylactoid.

● *Granulomatous diseases*, whether infective or non-infective, are associated with localized accumulations of activated macrophages which presumably are attempting to remove persistent antigen. Most commonly, a delayed (Type IV) hypersensitivity reaction is involved with lymphokine release causing macrophage attraction and activation. The macrophages then form epithelioid and giant cells. Sometimes, an immune complex (Type III) reaction is involved with complement activation and chemotaxis for macrophages. Tuberculosis is the classic example of an infective granulomatous disease. Non-infective types of granulomatous disease include foreign body reactions, hypersensitivity pneumonitis, carcinoid and Wegener's granulomatosis.

● *Pulmonary infiltrative diseases* may include elements of eosinophilia, vasculitis and fibrosis. A probable sequence in many forms of interstitial inflammation is the pulmonary deposition of circulating immune complexes, local activation of complement, recruitment of neutrophils and macrophages, and release of mediators and enzymes. Tissue damage then results and systemic features are common. Alveolitis may be classified as due to entrapment (e.g. fibrosing alveolitis) or as auto-immune (e.g. Goodpasture's syndrome). Vasculitis may be due to rheumatoid arthritis, systemic lupus erythematosus, polyarteritis or Wegener's granulomatosis. Fibrosis may be due to vasculitis, pneumoconiosis, granulomatosis or to non-immunological conditions such as haemosiderosis, paraquat, drugs, irradiation or chronic congestive cardiac failure.

Immunological investigations

There is a large array of laboratory immunological investigations and a great variety of techniques are available. Of these groups of tests, those measuring humoral factors (immunoglobulins, other serum protein, antibodies, complement components) are precise and their interpretation relatively clear-cut; those measuring cellular components (lymphocytes, phagocytes) are more variable and their interpretation more difficult; those measuring both humoral and cellular elements in vivo are also relatively difficult to standardize and their interpretation is limited. The investigations of most importance for respiratory medicine are summarized in Table 9.1.

Table 9.1. Immunological investigations

Immunoglobulins
   quantitative measurement
 Other proteins
   acute phase, coagulation,
   inhibitors, transport
 Specific antibody
   total IgE
   radioallergosorbent test
   precipitins
   skin tests
   nasal or bronchial challenge
 Auto-antibodies
   organ specific
   non-organ specific
	Complement
	   components
	   inhibitors
	 Immune complexes
	   direct assay
	 Lymphocytes
	   total number
	   T and B cells, T cell subsets
	   skin tests
	   functional tests
	 Phagocytes
	   total number (neutrophils, monocytes)
	   functional tests

Asthma

Definition

Bronchial asthma is currently defined as recurrent, reversible, generalized airways obstruction, associated with increased bronchial reactivity. The definition of asthma has been the subject of much controversy over the years, which is hardly surprising since its aetiology remains unknown and since clinically it overlaps other conditions associated with airways obstruction.

Epidemiology

There is an overall incidence, or cumulative prevalence, of overt asthma in most countries of 1−5%. In addition, the incidence of wheezy bronchitis in children and of increased bronchial reactivity at all ages appears to be up to 10% or more. Thus, about 10% of the population either has or has had asthma or has an asthmatic tendency.

Although asthma can occur at any age, there are two peaks of incidence, one in early childhood and another in middle life. In young children, asthma is about one and a half times more common in boys. Many children with asthma show substantial clinical improvement by the age of 12 years, although increased bronchial reactivity tends to persist. Patients with late-onset asthma have a poorer prognosis in that the disease is often more severe, less reversible, more steroid-dependent and much less likely to remit.

By contrast with its substantial morbidity, asthma has had a low mortality, especially since the introduction of cortico-steroids over 30 years ago. The average mortality rate is now about 2−4 per 100000 population per year. Disturbingly, however, this mortality still includes a number of young people who are seemingly not severely asthmatic but who die unexpectedly during an acute, fulminating attack.

Genetic factors are important in predisposing to asthma, since a positive family history is common, especially in asthma that is extrinsic or associated with atopy. However, the exact mode of inheritance is obscure. In monozygotic twins, concordance for asthma is only about 20% and in dizygotic twins, only about 5%.

Types of asthma

Asthma is a clinical label encompassing a number of different entities which are related to a varying degree.

- *'Extrinsic' asthma* is the more common and perhaps the most classical type. This unsatisfactory term implies that the stimulus arises from the environment, usually in the form of an allergen. This type of asthma is the one usually seen in childhood, is associated with atopy, has a familial predisposition, and tends to respond well to therapy and usually to remit after a few years.
- *'Intrinsic' asthma* is the other main type. It was so named (or rather misnamed) because the stimuli were thought not to arise externally. This type of asthma is the one usually arising in later life, is not associated with atopy, is often associated with infection, and tends to be more difficult to treat and not to remit. Better terms nowadays than extrinsic and intrinsic are childhood-onset or allergic and late-onset or idiopathic.
- *'Wheezy bronchitis'* is the term used to describe the condition in children of episodic chest infection associated with wheeze. The vast majority of these children have bronchial asthma and wheezy bronchitis has been used as a euphemism, perhaps to avoid frightening parents with a 'more serious' diagnosis.
- *'Asthmatic bronchitis'* refers to another intermediate condition in which chronic, or sometimes acute, bronchitis is associated with prominent wheeze. Although such patients have predominant bronchitis, the term is not unreasonable since there is often a useful response to bronchodilators.
- *Exercise-induced asthma* is not a separate entity, since most asthmatic patients are prone to exacerbations during most types of physical exertion, particularly in cold weather. However, in some patients it is their only symptomatic type of asthma.
- *Status asthmaticus* refers to an acute episode which is prolonged, refractory to simple therapy, and usually requires hospitalization.
- *'Cardiac' asthma* is the old term describing the association of wheeze with acute pulmonary congestion and oedema due to left heart failure. Since there is a degree of reversible endobronchial obstruction present, the term is not unreasonable, although of course the treatment is mostly quite different.
- *Latent asthma* describes clinically normal subjects who have increased bronchial reactivity. They may have a past history or family history of asthma. It is possible that some of these subjects may later suffer overt asthma, depending on the intensity of the stimulus to which they may be exposed.
- *Occupational asthma* occurs in many people exposed to environmental agents such as isocyanates, wood and grain dusts, animal products, enzymes and soldering fluxes. Many of these effects are due to hypersensitivity and often occur in previously atopic subjects.
- *Asthma-like symptoms* can, in fact, develop in any normal subject given a severe enough stimulus, such as many toxic gases. The presence of a viral infection heightens the susceptibility of normal subjects as well as asthmatics to such stimuli.

Since anyone can develop asthma-like symptoms given a sufficient stimulus, it is therefore clearly important that the definition of clinical asthma includes the concept of abnormally increased bronchial reactivity.

● *Eosinophilia with fleeting pulmonary infiltrates* is associated with asthma in hypersensitivity to the fungus, *Aspergillus fumigatus*, and in polyarteritis nodosa. *Carcinoid tumour*, particularly with liver metastases, may give rise to asthmatic symptoms and *pulmonary embolism* is classically associated with wheeze in some patients, even to the extent of mimicking asthma.

Pathogenesis

The pathogenesis of asthma is incompletely understood but appears to include immunological reactions, release of chemical mediators and probably reflex events (Fig. 10.1).

The immediate (Type I) mainly IgE-associated immunological reaction to antigen has been considered of major relevance in many asthmatic responses, especially in atopy. The immediate hypersensitivity reaction is associated with the release of a variety of chemical mediators, including histamine, leucotrienes, eosinophilic chemotactic factor of anaphylaxis (ECF-A) and platelet-activating factor (PAF) (all from mast cells) and prostaglandins and bradykinin. Many mediators also require vagal reflexes for their full effect. These reactions can be suppressed by cromoglycate but not by corticosteroids. The cytotoxic (Type II) immunological reaction has not been implicated in asthma. The late (Type III) mainly IgG-associated immunological reaction to antigen gives rise to local immune

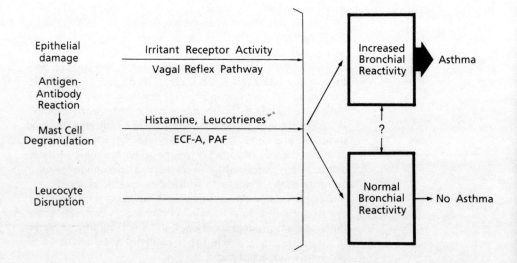

Fig. 10.1. Pathogenesis of bronchial asthma. A variety of mechanisms may lead to release of substances producing airway narrowing. However, asthma arises only in those persons who in addition have increased bronchial reactivity.

complex formation and complement activation, also with release of mediators, such as histamine. These reactions have been implicated in delayed-onset asthmatic responses. They can be suppressed by corticosteroids but not by cromoglycate. The delayed (Type IV) cell-mediated immunological reaction with release of lymphokines may be of relevance in some asthmatic responses, such as in allergic aspergillosis.

The net result of these pathogenetic mechanisms is bronchial smooth muscle contraction (bronchospasm), mucosal oedema and lumenal plugging with viscid mucus (Fig.10.2). These three factors are jointly responsible for the airways obstruction in asthma.

Clinical features

The main symptoms of asthma are episodic dyspnoea and wheeze. Difficulty is experienced chiefly with expiration, which is prolonged. Cough is frequent, even without associated chest infection. Sometimes small amounts of viscid mucus or plugs may be coughed up. The sputum may be purulent, due either to its eosinophil content or to endobronchial infection.

The history will reveal the frequency and duration of attacks, including any seasonal pattern, the clinical state between attacks, previous and current therapy, and the past and family history, including atopy. In particular, the history may eluci-

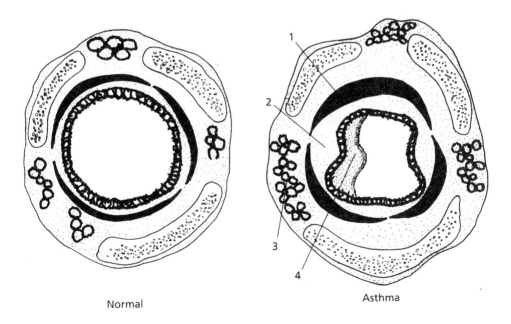

Normal

Asthma

Fig. 10.2. Airway pathology in bronchial asthma. In contrast to the normal situation (left), there is bronchial smooth muscle contraction (1), mucosal oedema (2), mucous gland hypertrophy (3) and intralumenal secretions (4).

date the responsible precipitating factor — allergen (especially house dust, animal dander, fungi, pollens, aspirin, foods), infection, psychological stress or non-specific agents, such as exercise, cold air or environmental pollutant.

Physical examination between attacks may be entirely normal. In the symptomatic patient, and even in some asymptomatic patients, airways obstruction is apparent with audible wheeze, prolonged expiration and rhonchi on auscultation. The lungs are hyperinflated, the accessory muscles of respiration are in use and the patient is clearly in distress. In very severe obstruction, wheeze decreases and the chest may even become silent — an ominous sign. Pulsus paradoxus also indicates the presence of severe obstruction, as does tachycardia and central cyanosis.

Investigations

Lung function tests

In the diagnosis and management of asthma, simple spirometric lung function tests have a key role, similar to that of the sphygmomanometer in the management of hypertension. PEF measurements are a somewhat less satisfactory substitute but because of their simplicity they are ideal for bedside assessment and the keeping of records by patients.

In symptomatic asthma, the FEV_1 and FEV_1/VC ratio are reduced; in more severe obstruction the VC is also decreased but not by as much as the FEV_1; like the FEV_1, the MMEFR and PEF are similarly reduced. The reversibility of airways obstruction should always be formally assessed. If the FEV_1 is significantly decreased, spirometry should be repeated after inhaled bronchodilator, such as isoprenaline or salbutamol, when an increase of 15% or more is evidence of reversibility.

In association with the obstructed pattern of ventilatory capacity, lung volume measurements show hyperinflation with increased RV, FRC and TLC. Lung mechanics show increased airway resistance and increased lung compliance. The distribution of ventilation is uneven and ventilation/blood flow relations are disturbed. Gas transfer is usually normal. The arterial oxygen tension is decreased; the arterial carbon dioxide tension is decreased in mild to moderate asthma but increased in severe, prolonged asthma.

Similar changes may be found in many asymptomatic patients, reflecting the insensitivity of the patient's own perception of the severity of his asthma. Some 20% of asthmatics have poor perception of this nature.

If there is no current obstruction in an asymptomatic patient with suspected asthma, bronchial reactivity may be assessed by spirometry before and after bronchial provocation with inhaled methacholine or histamine, or with exercise. As with the bronchodilator response, a change of 15% or more is indicative of enhanced reactivity, though more sophisticated calculations of indices of bronchial reactivity are now commonly made.

In patients with severe asthma, the only lung function test

which can be performed, and which is appropriate, is arterial blood gas analysis.

In all patients with asthma, serial lung function tests are important in following progress, assessing therapy, relating symptoms to function and documenting peaks and troughs of obstruction. An index of asthma instability is an increased diurnal variation in obstruction as detected, for example, by serial measurements of PEF.

Chest X-ray

The chest X-ray is usually normal, even in acute asthma, except for hyperinflation. The chief value of the routine chest X-ray in acute asthma is to exclude pneumothorax and sometimes to demonstrate consolidation due to infection or segmental collapse due to mucus plugging.

Laboratory tests

Sputum examination may show the presence of many eosinophils, especially in macroscopically purulent specimens. Charcot–Leyden crystals (fragmented and coalesced eosinophils) and Curschmann's spirals (bronchiolar casts) may be seen. Microscopic examination and appropriate culture for bacteria and fungi should be made.

Full blood examination should be performed to detect the presence of eosinophilia.

Suspected allergens are best identified by skin prick tests or sometimes by bronchial challenge. Radioallergosorbent tests (RAST) for specific allergens usually add little further information and considerable extra cost. Total IgE measurement may sometimes be helpful, although it mainly indicates that the subject is atopic.

Diagnosis

The diagnosis is usually established on clinical grounds and should be confirmed by the demonstration on lung function testing of either reversible airways obstruction or increased bronchial reactivity. The most difficult differential diagnosis is usually from bronchitis but, as indicated earlier, there may be considerable overlap between the two conditions and the distinction may be more semantic than real.

Treatment

The management of asthma is largely symptomatic, in that there is no present way of normalizing the underlying bronchial hyper-reactivity. However, modern drug therapy can offer most patients good symptomatic control as well as normal interval function. Some trial and adjustment of therapy is often necessary before a satisfactory regimen is reached which will control the various situations encountered in an individual patient.

The drugs used include sympathomimetics, theophylline compounds, anticholinergics, cromglycate and corticosteroids. Sympathomimetics currently preferred are those with relatively selective β_2 agonist properties, including orciprenaline (metaproterenol), salbutamol (albuterol), terbutaline and fenoterol. These drugs are best given by inhalation (metered aerosol or nebulizer), though parenteral and oral preparations are also available. Theophylline is given as aminophylline intravenously or rectally, or theophylline orally. The anticholinergic agent, ipratropium bromide, has recently become available and is used by inhalation. Cromoglycate modulates mediator release

Table 10.1. Drugs used in asthma

Medication	Formulation	Strength	Dosage
β₂ agonists			
Orciprenaline	metered aerosol	0.075 mg/actuation	0.150 mg 8 hrly
(Metaproterenol)	nebulized aerosol	2 mg/ml	1 ml 6 hrly
	tablet	20 mg	20 mg 6–8 hrly
	syrup	10 mg/5 ml	20 mg 6–8 hrly
	injection	0.5 mg/ml	0.5–1 mg i.m. or i.v.
Salbutamol	metered aerosol	0.1 mg/actuation	0.2 mg 4–6 hrly
(Albuterol)	nebulized aerosol	5 mg/ml	0.5 ml 6 hrly
	dry inhalation	0.2 mg/capsule	0.2 mg 6 hrly
	tablet	4 mg	4–8 mg 6 hrly
	syrup	2 mg/5 ml	5–10 ml 6 hrly
	injection	0.5 mg/ml	0.5 mg s.c./i.m. 4 hrly
			0.25 mg i.v. over 1 min
			5–20 μg/min i.v. infusion
Terbutaline	metered aerosol	0.25 mg/actuation	0.5 mg 4–6 hrly
	nebulized aerosol	10 mg/ml	0.5 ml 6 hrly
	tablet	5 mg	2.5–5 mg 8 hrly
	injection	0.1 & 0.5 mg/ml	0.25 mg s.c. 6 hrly
Fenoterol	metered aerosol	0.25 mg/actuation	0.5 mg 4–6 hrly
	nebulized aerosol	10 mg/ml	0.5 ml 6 hrly
	tablet	2.5 mg	2.5–5 mg 8 hrly
	injection	0.1 & 0.5 mg/ml	0.25 mg s.c. 8 hrly
Corticosteroids			
Beclomethasone	metered aerosol	0.05 mg/actuation	up to 1 mg daily
diproprionate	dry inhalation	0.1 mg capsule	up to 1 mg daily
Prednisolone	tablet	1 & 5 mg	various regimens—
Betamethasone	tablet	0.5 mg	acute, intermittent
			or long-term low-dose
Hydrocortisone	injection	100 & 250 mg/ml	100–250 mg bolus i.v.
sodium succinate			500 mg daily i.v. infusion
Other drugs			
Aminophylline	tablet	100 mg	100–300 mg 6 hrly
	injection	25 mg/ml	4–6 mg/kg i.v. then
			0.5 mg/kg/hr i.v.
Theophylline	tablet	various	500–1200 mg daily
preparations	elixir	strengths	(high-dose or longterm
	suppositories		theophylline therapy
			should be monitored with
			blood levels)
Sodium	dry inhalation	20 mg capsule	80–160 mg daily
cromoglycate	metered aerosol	1 mg/actuation	8–16 mg daily
	nebulized aerosol	20 mg/2 ml	20 mg 6 hrly
Ipratropium	metered aerosol	0.02 mg/actuation	0.04 mg 6 hrly
bromide	nebulized aerosol	0.25 mg/ml	1–2 ml 6 hrly

from mast cells and is not generally in itself a bronchodilator. It is used solely for prophylaxis and is given by inhalation. Corticosteroids are given intravenously, orally or by metered aerosol. Common doses of these drugs are indicated in Table 10.1.

The general principles of the drug treatment of asthma are outlined in Table 10.2. Acute attacks require sympathomimetics and theophylline. Corticosteroids are used if asthma is very severe; increased doses are required if the patient is already receiving maintenance doses of this drug. The dose and route of therapy are determined by the severity of the acute episode. Very severe asthma needs hospitalization and treatment for respiratory failure.

Chronic asthma requires continued sympathomimetics and usually concomitant therapy, such as theophylline, ipratropium, cromoglycate and/or corticosteroids. Unless the patient has normal lung function as well as no symptoms, such treatment should be maintained during the interval state. Periodic clinical and functional review is important but often tends to be overlooked. Other therapeutic considerations include treatment of an infective precipitating factor, possible 'desensitization' in house dust mite allergy, avoidance of known ag-

	Asthma assessment	Drug regimen
Table 10.2. An outline of drug therapy in asthma	Mild & intermittent	β_2 agonist aerosol (perhaps intermittently)
	Mild & chronic	β_2 agonist aerosol & Sodium cromoglycate &/or Beclomethasone diproprionate &/or Ipratropium bromide (all used regularly) Oral corticosteroids (short course over 7–10 days for acute exacerbations)
	Severe & chronic	β_2 agonist by nebulizer system & Oral corticosteroids & Beclomethasone diproprionate & Oral theophylline & Ipratropium bromide
	Severe & acute	β_2 agonist by nebulizer system & Parenteral aminophylline & Parenteral hydrocortisone & Oxygen (consider patient-administered adrenaline kit)
	Severe with anaphylaxis	Parenteral adrenaline & Oxygen & Parenteral hydrocortisone & Parenteral promethazine

gravating factors including environmental pollutants, irritants and allergens, and psychological support.

Prognosis

In perhaps no other condition is appropriate education of the patient more important. An understanding of the general nature of asthma should produce better compliance with any therapeutic plan, better cooperation in the avoidance of known trigger factors, and prevention of a relentless search for a 'cure'. Asthma is compatible with a long and active life, with in most cases minimal disruption of life-style. However, a significant mortality rate remains and in some cases death seems neither entirely predictable nor preventable.

11   Chronic Bronchitis and Emphysema

Introduction

Diffuse chronic airways obstruction (CAO) is the most frequent and important respiratory problem in both advanced and developing societies. Chronic obstructive pulmonary disease (COPD) or chronic obstructive lung disease (COLD) are frequently used as global terms for this group of conditions but such nomenclature has the disadvantage that it tries to embrace several specific and quite different disorders under a single umbrella. These disorders are chiefly chronic bronchitis and emphysema. However, they merge not only into each other but also into both asthma (when there is associated bronchial hyper-reactivity) and bronchiectasis (when there is some associated localized, large bronchial dilatation and destruction).

- *Chronic bronchitis* is defined clinically as the presence of cough and sputum on most days during at least three consecutive months for more than two successive years (provided other chronic infections such as major bronchiectasis and tuberculosis have been excluded).
- *Emphysema* is defined pathologically as dilatation and destruction of air spaces distal to the terminal bronchiole.

Epidemiology

The prevalence of chronic bronchitis and emphysema has been difficult to establish because of their gradual development, variable definitions and population differences. Surveys have shown that 7–31% of the population have some degree of chronic airways obstruction, depending on age, sex, smoking habit, occupation and urbanization. Chronic airways obstruction is the single largest cause of loss of working days and its overall socioeconomic burden is vast.

The long-term prognosis, based mainly on older studies, is poor, particularly if the FEV_1 is less than 1 litre or if there is hypercapnia or cor pulmonale. The five year mortality is about 50% in symptomatic patients. Mortality is about 10% per year when the FEV_1 is 1 litre and the FEV_1 declines on average by about 100 ml per year.

Mortality rates show great international variation and there is clearly considerable variation in medical death certification of these diseases. The mortality from all forms of chronic airways obstruction has ranged from 70–120 per 100 000 population among men in Great Britain. Mortality is greater in men, in older patients, in urban areas and in winter. Since the late 1960s, there appears to have been a progressive decline in mortality from chronic airways obstruction, perhaps related to reduced smoking and atmospheric pollution.

Aetiology

A number of factors are presumed to cause chronic bronchitis and emphysema although their relative importance remains unclear. Tobacco smoking, atmospheric pollution and infection are the three most prominent factors, together with hereditary α_1-antitrypsin deficiency in some cases of emphysema. Although the majority of patients with chronic bronchitis have at least some emphysema, and vice versa, the reasons for the different diseases from similar causative factors are unclear. Chronic cough and sputum may initially be induced by inhaled noxious substances (cigarette smoke and environmental pollutants), and subsequent acute and eventually chronic infection becomes then more likely. Certainly a change in the biochemical nature of bronchial secretions seems to be an early marker of developing bronchitis. The alveolar destruction in emphysema may be caused by the release of proteases from damaged leucocytes. What remains completely unresolved is why different individuals exposed to seemingly comparable insults respond so differently, some with chronic bronchitis and/or emphysema of varying severity and many with little or no disability at all.

Pathology

• In *chronic bronchitis*, the chief site of pathological change is in the conducting airways. There is an increase in the size and number of mucus glands in the bronchial walls. There may also be a significant increase in goblet cell numbers. Airways obstruction is due to thickening of bronchial walls and narrowing of the bronchial lumen, together with excessive intralumenal secretions. Bronchial smooth muscle is hypertrophied in those patients with associated wheeze. The small airways are particularly affected in early chronic bronchitis, with inflammation of the walls, squamous metaplasia and excessive mucus secretion. Many of these changes are induced by smoking and are potentially reversible. The inflammatory component may be important in maintaining and increasing airflow obstruction.

• In *emphysema*, the chief site of pathological change is in the terminal respiratory units or parenchyma. Two main types of emphysema are recognized (Fig. 11.1). In centrilobular emphysema, the centre of the lobule is affected. There is associated chronic bronchiolitis and the process is more marked at the apices. In panlobular or panacinar emphysema, uniform destruction of the entire lobule occurs with severe architectural disruption. Widespread panlobular emphysema is not common, except in α_1-antitrypsin deficiency. The relation between the two types of emphysema is unresolved, though the two can coexist and the former may sometimes progress to the latter.

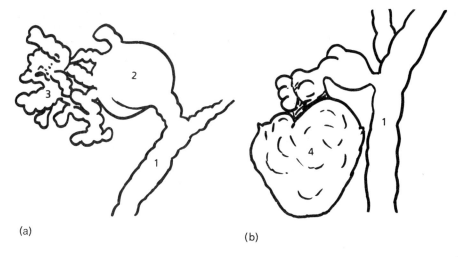

(a)

(b)

Fig. 11.1. Emphysema with dilatation and destruction distal to the terminal bronchiole (1). In centrilobular emphysema (a), proximal parts of the lobule are chiefly affected (2) with relative preservation of distal alveoli (3). In panacinar emphysema (b), the entire acinus is affected (4).

Emphysema gives rise to airways obstruction primarily because of airway collapse during expiration due to loss of surrounding tissue support and thus of elastic recoil. The loss of elastic tissue is a notable feature in emphysema and probably indicates that agents with a strong elastase activity act locally in its development. Other forms of emphysema occur with dilatation alone and no destruction or inflammation and thus without airway obstruction. Such forms occur as compensation for loss of lung tissue, irregularly in the vicinity of scars and following local ball-valve bronchial obstruction.

Clinical features

The chief symptoms of *chronic bronchitis* are, as its definition requires, cough and sputum. These are most marked initially in the morning. These symptoms may have progressed almost imperceptibly from a 'smoker's cough', probably with exacerbations during respiratory tract infections. The sputum is mucopurulent except during an acute exacerbation when it is more frankly purulent. The patient is prone to such infections which usually originate with an acute viral upper respiratory tract infection. Persistent purulent sputum suggests associated bronchiectasis. Large quantities of frothy, serous secretions (bronchorrhoea) sometimes occur when there is gross mucus gland hypertrophy. Wheeze, especially on exertion, is noted by many patients. Dyspnoea occurs in more advanced disease and is mainly exertional. Nocturnal dyspnoea with orthopnoea is also seen in patients in whom significant tracheobronchial secretions accumulate during sleep, giving rise to a sequence of progressive obstruction, awakening and dyspnoea, followed

99/*Chronic Bronchitis and Emphysema*

by sitting up, productive coughing and improvement. This sequence may not always be easy to distinguish from the paroxysmal nocturnal dyspnoea of acute pulmonary oedema. Hypoxaemia, polycythaemia, cyanosis, chronic hypercapnia and cor pulmonale with marked peripheral oedema are typical in more severe disease, though they may be present for many years. The patient showing this constellation of features has been picturesquely referred to as a 'blue bloater' (or type B).

The chief symptom of *emphysema* is dyspnoea. This becomes progressively more severe until exertional tolerance may be so poor that the patient has difficulty even speaking or dressing. Expiration is difficult and prolonged, and pursed lip breathing may be used to limit airway collapse during expiration by maintaining a slightly positive airway pressure. Loss of weight is common. Cough and sputum are not typical. Respiratory failure and cor pulmonale occur only as relatively terminal events. By contrast, the patient showing this constellation of features has been referred to as a 'pink puffer' (or type A).

Physical examination may reveal a wasted patient, especially in the later stages of emphysema. Plethora and central cyanosis indicate the presence of respiratory failure, which is usually chronic. Clubbing is rare and never marked unless there is associated carcinoma. Examination of the chest shows hyperinflation, especially in emphysema. The accessory muscles of respiration are used in advanced disease and there is evidence of wide intrapleural pressure swings, as the subclavicular and suprasternal fossae draw in during inspiration and the jugular venous pressure rises during expiration. The lungs are hyperresonant, breath sounds are generally decreased and widespread rhonchi are prominent, especially during expiration. Evidence of cor pulmonale includes right ventricular heave on palpation and gallop on auscultation, raised jugular venous pressure, hepatomegaly and peripheral oedema. The liver may appear to be enlarged even in the absence of cor pulmonale but this is due to diaphragmatic flattening and in this case the liver is not tender.

The clinical features of pure emphysema and pure chronic bronchitis are not commonly seen, since as previously indicated, most patients have mixed disease on pathological, functional and clinical grounds. The chief virtue of the separate descriptions is as an instructive exercise to describe the two ends of the spectrum of chronic airways obstruction, rather than to fit each patient into one or other category exclusively. However, the relative contribution by each process influences prognosis and is worth assessing.

Investigations

Lung function tests

Since chronic bronchitis is defined on clinical grounds and emphysema on pathological grounds, it is not surprising that functional abnormalities do not necessarily correlate with the clinicopathological changes in either condition. The general pattern, however, is one of airways obstruction, readily demonstrable by spirometry. There is reduced FEV_1 and

FEV$_1$/VC ratio; the VC is also decreased in advanced disease, though not by as much as the FEV$_1$; the MMEFR and PEF are decreased concomitantly with the FEV$_1$. Typically, there is little or no response to bronchodilator. The earliest changes that can be detected are those of small airways disease, with reduced MMEFR, reduced flow rate at low lung volume and increase frequency dependence of compliance.

In chronic bronchitis, there tends to be no absolute hyperinflation, so that the TLC is normal despite an increased RV. Compliance is normal, as is gas transfer. There is hypoxaemia with or without hypercapnia. Cardiac output is normal, pulmonary vascular resistance is increased and pulmonary artery pressures are increased.

In emphysema, there is often striking hyperinflation with an increased TLC as well as RV. Compliance is increased and gas transfer decreased. Arterial blood gas values are relatively well preserved. Cardiac output tends to be low, so that although pulmonary vascular resistance is increased, pulmonary artery pressures are relatively normal.

The chief difference between chronic bronchitis and emphysema may be due to differences in respiratory drive (possibly genetically based) rather than to differences in pathology or pathophysiology. Thus, the patient with emphysema has a well preserved respiratory drive and attempts to maintain normal blood gases, even at the expense of a substantially increased workload. By contrast, the patient with chronic bronchitis has a 'lazy' respiratory drive and 'gives in' to the increased workload, but at the expense of abnormal blood gases. Other variables such as pulmonary vasoconstriction may also contribute to the different patterns of dysfunction.

The most useful tests for clinical purposes are:
- *spirometry* to assess the severity of disease, its long-term progression and its acute exacerbations.
- *gas transfer* to suggest the amount of emphysema.
- *arterial blood gases* to indicate the degree of respiratory failure.

Chest X-ray

The chest X-ray in chronic bronchitis and emphysema is not diagnostic and often not even characteristic. In chronic bronchitis it is often normal. Thickened bronchial walls ('tram lines') radiating from the hila may sometimes be identified, although this is arguable. Pulmonary artery dilatation may be seen in cor pulmonale. In emphysema, again little radiological change may be evident even in advanced disease, although hyperinflation, patchy translucency and diaphragmatic depression are more typical.

The chief value of the chest X-ray is in detecting a number of complications, such as consolidation, bullae or pneumothorax.

Laboratory investigations

The main laboratory investigations of value are microbiological examination of sputum, haematological assessment for

101/*Chronic Bronchitis and Emphysema*

polycythaemia and perhaps for neutrophilia or eosinophilia, and biochemical measurement of the serum α_1-antitrypsin level.

Management

Prevention

It is likely that much chronic bronchitis and emphysema is preventable given the aetiological factors involved. Indeed, reduction in smoking and atmospheric pollution and better attention to respiratory infections have probably already contributed to the significant decrease in morbidity and mortality from chronic airways obstruction in recent times. Even in patients with established disease, reduction in these factors has been shown to halt progression of disease.

Symptomatic

1 Smoking should be stopped.
2 Bronchodilator therapy is frequently helpful, even in patients who do not show objective improvement in spirometric indices following a single dose of inhaled bronchodilator in the laboratory. The appropriate regimen is similar to that for asthma and includes sympathomimetics, theophylline and anticholinergics. Cromoglycate is rarely of value. Occasional patients respond well to corticosteroids and a trial is often worthwhile.
3 Mucolytic or expectorant drugs have not been shown to be of value.
4 Antibiotics may be given long-term to decrease the incidence of infective exacerbations. Although this goal has been shown to be feasible, long-term improvement in lung function has not been demonstrated. In most patients, it is probably simpler, cheaper and more logical to treat acute infectious exacerbations promptly as they occur with an appropriate antibiotic such as amoxycillin.
5 Physiotherapy in the form of breathing exercises and postural drainage may be of help to some patients. More particularly, exercise training has been found to be of dramatic benefit for some patients.
6 Long-term oxygen therapy at low flow rates for at least 12 hours/day has been shown to reduce cor pulmonale, improve symptoms and increase longevity.
7 Psychosocial support, including vocational retraining, is an important measure for many patients. Rehabilitation is often effective but requires patient confidence and motivation.

Complications

• *Acute respiratory failure* requires hospitalization and specific management. Admission to an acute care facility is desirable provided the patient's condition is seriously compromised but has some potential reversibility.
• *Cor pulmonale* is treated with diuretics but digitalis should be used with caution. The unexpected onset of cor pulmonale should raise the suspicion of pulmonary thromboembolism. However, this diagnosis can be difficult to confirm as the lung scan will usually be grossly abnormal anyway.
• Localized large *bullae* may occasionally warrant surgical resection.

12   Respiratory Infections

Introduction

Respiratory infections are the commonest of all infections. The most serious respiratory infection, pneumonia, carries the highest mortality of all infections diseases and is the fifth leading cause of death.

Table 12.1. Respiratory defence mechanisms

Nasopharynx
Cough
Mucus blanket & ciliary motion
Antimicrobial substances in secretions:
  non-specific (e.g. lysozyme)
  specific (e.g. IgA)
Alveolar macrophages
Systemic factors:
  IgG, T lymphocytes,
  neutrophils, complement

The chief respiratory defence mechanisms against infection are listed in Table 12.1. The first three mechanisms have been referred to as first-line defences and the last three as second-line defences.

When one or more of these defences fail, respiratory infection may result, usually via one of the following three routes:

1 *Inhalation of aerosolized droplets.* This has been the best understood mechanism of respiratory infection and it applies to viruses, mycobacteria, fungi and some pneumococci.

2 *Aspiration of pharyngeal secretions.* This has recently become recognized as a major mechanism of lower respiratory tract infection and it applies to most bacteria. Aspiration of small amounts of nasopharyngeal and oropharyngeal secretions has been shown to occur during sleep even in normal subjects. Aspiration becomes important quantitatively when there is a depressed conscious state or upper gastrointestinal disease, and qualitatively when there is oral sepsis. The resultant infection is often a subtle microbiological problem, sometimes chronic and indolent, and is associated with colonization of the lower respiratory tract with mixed oral flora. When aspiration occurs in hospital patients whose oral flora contains Gram-negative bacilli or staphylococci, more serious infection may follow.

3 *Haematogenous spread*. This occurs in bacteraemia or fungaemia. It applies particularly to Gram-negative bacilli and also staphylococci.

The natural history of pneumonia nowadays tends to be modified by a variety of factors, including previous antibiotic therapy, hospitalization, chronic lung disease, and systemic disorders and their treatment. Thus, more varied pathogens and particularly nosocomial and opportunistic infections are increasingly seen. The major respiratory pathogens are listed in Table 12.2.

Table 12.2. Major respiratory pathogens

Gram-positive cocci
pneumococcus, *Streptococcus pyogenes,*
Staphylococcus aureus
Gram-negative bacilli
klebsiella, *E.coli*, pseudomonas, proteus,
serratia, enterobacter, acinetobacter
bacteroides
legionella
Gram-negative cocci
meningococcus
Gram-positive bacilli
Gram-negative cocco-bacilli
Haemophilus influenzae, B. catarrhalis
Mixed flora
Mycobacteria
Protozoa
pneumocystis
Fungi
Mycoplasma
Chlamydia
Coxiella
Viruses
influenza, parainfluenza, adeno, rhino,
respiratory syncytial, varicella/zoster, CMV

Upper respiratory tract infection

Upper respiratory tract infections (URTIs) are among the commonest afflictions of mankind at all ages. Most are due to viruses or haemophilus and include pharyngitis, obstructive laryngitis (croup) and influenza-like illness, as well as the common cold (coryza). Apart from the emergencies related to croup and epiglottitis and to the occasional severe respiratory and circulatory complications of influenza, URTIs are chiefly of major clinical significance in those patients in whom secondary bacterial infection of the lower respiratory tract follows.

Acute tracheitis and bronchitis

Acute tracheitis or bronchitis is usually due to infection with *Streptococcus pneumoniae* or *Haemophilus influenzae*. Acute tracheitis is manifested by irritating cough and retrosternal discomfort, and acute bronchitis by cough, purulent sputum, sometimes dyspnoea and wheeze, and coarse crackles. In both, the chest X-ray remains normal. Acute bronchitis is preferably treated with an antibiotic, such as amoxycillin.

Classical bacterial pneumonia

Classical bacterial pneumonia is subdivided according to the causative organism and the anatomical site involved. The most common bacteria involved are *Streptococcus pneumoniae*, *Staphylococcus aureus*, *Klebsiella pneumoniae*, other aerobic Gram-negative bacilli (e.g. *E. coli, Pseudomonas aeruginosa*), anaerobic Gram-negative bacilli (e.g. *Bacteroides sp.*), and other streptococci. Sometimes, pneumonia may occur as part of a specific bacterial disease (e.g. pertussis, anthrax, plague). The causative organism can usually be identified, provided antibiotics have not already been given.

• *Lobar pneumonia* is most commonly pneumococcal, though other bacteria, particularly *Staphylococcus aureus* and *Klebsiella pneumoniae*, can also cause similar extensive consolidation. Lobar pneumonia may also be caused by *Haemophilus influenzae* in the elderly or debilitated, or by legionella in some community-acquired cases.

• *Bronchopneumonia* which involves lobules and is usually bilateral may be caused by most organisms.

• *Segmental or subsegmental pneumonia* is common in patients with severe or prolonged URTIs associated with cough and may represent aspiration of infected mucus without major bacterial colonization.

The clinical features of bacterial pneumonia classically comprise fever, cough and sputum which is purulent and sometimes rusty. The onset is relatively rapid though there is commonly a preceding event such as an URTI, exposure to cold or anaesthesia, or alcoholic excess. There is commonly pleuritic pain and sometimes herpes labialis. On examination, the patient is febrile and ill with tachypnoea, tachycardia and often cyanosis. The affected part of the lung has less air entry and is dull to percussion, and there is bronchial breathing with increased vocal fremitus and resonance. Crackles are usual and a pleuritic rub may be heard. The clinical features of segmental or subsegmental pneumonia are minor.

Chest X-ray shows a relatively uniform density with an air bronchogram in the area of lung involved. The development of abscess cavities is typical of staphylococcal or klebsiella pneumonia. Arterial blood gas analysis is required if respiratory failure is suspected. Haematological examination shows a considerable leucocytosis with a marked neutrophilia and the erythrocyte sedimentation rate (ESR) is high.

Microbiological examination of sputum is clearly the key to identifying the specific aetiological organism, but an informed clinical guess is often surprisingly accurate. Many organisms isolated from sputum, even in cases of overt pneumonia, are unlikely major aetiological agents (such as *Streptococcus viridans* and upper respiratory tract flora). Since expectorated sputum is always contaminated with oropharyngeal flora, microscopy of Gram-stained preparations is the most important part of sputum examination. Multiple pathogens may sometimes be identified in sputum. Blood cultures are often positive in severe pneumonia and may reveal an organism which has not been able to be identified in sputum.

The diagnosis of pneumonia is not usually difficult. However, it may not always be easy to establish the specific aetiological organism or to separate the extent of an acute process from underlying disease, such as chronic airways obstruction or carcinoma.

Treatment is with appropriate chemotherapy and hospitalization is required for all but milder cases. Penicillin in large doses remains the antibiotic of choice for pneumococcal pneumonia. For seriously ill patients, doses of up to 14 g (24 mega units) per day of benzyl penicillin should be given intravenously. For less seriously ill patients, lower doses intramuscularly are adequate. Staphylococcal pneumonia should be treated with β-lactamase resistant penicillin, such as flucloxacillin, in doses of 2−8 g per day in the seriously ill. Aerobic Gram-negative organisms should usually be treated with an aminoglycoside, such as gentamicin (80 mg 8 hourly intravenously or intramuscularly), and anaerobes with metronidazole (500 mg 8 hourly intravenously) or clindamycin (1.2 g 12 hourly intravenously or intramuscularly). In general, for more seriously ill patients, larger doses and broader cover need to be given, preferably intravenously, and for less seriously ill patients, lower doses, either intramuscularly or orally. Amoxycillin, cotrimoxazole, cephalosporins (especially third generation agents such as cefotaxime) and new extended-spectrum penicillins (such as ticarcillin, piperacillin, mezlocillin) offer effective chemotherapy for many respiratory infections but their use should be based on laboratory evidence, known local antibiotic sensitivity patterns or the advice of a medical microbiologist.

In pneumococcal pneumonia a response to therapy should be seen within 24 hours but in pneumonia due to klebsiella it may take some days, and in staphylococcal pneumonia it may take even longer. A delayed response should suggest that the identification of the organism or the choice of antibiotic is wrong or the general diagnosis itself is in error. Treatment should generally continue well past the resolution of fever and usually for 7−10 days. Lobar pneumonia and bronchopneumonia are treated similarly. Segmental or subsegmental pneumonia does not usually require therapy in its own right, though a course of oral amoxycillin is reasonable if symptoms persist.

General aspects of management include oxygen, fluid replacement and analgesics. Seriously ill patients should be admitted to an acute care area where there are facilities for resuscitation, intravenous management, endotracheal intubation and mechanical ventilation if necessary.

Complications of severe pneumonia include pleural effusion, empyema, pneumothorax, lung abscess, septicaemia, metastatic abscess formation, circulatory failure, disseminated intravascular coagulation and, rarely, acute adrenal insufficiency (Waterhouse−Friderichsen syndrome).

The prognosis of even severe pneumonia nowadays is good, except where it complicates other major illness (including influenza) or occurs in frail patients. Residual disability is uncommon, except where underlying respiratory disease is present. Poorly resolving or recurrent pneumonia should prompt a search for resistant organisms, abscess, tuberculosis, carcinoma, anatomical abnormality or an immunological abnormality. An anatomical abnormality is suggested when infection recurs in the same bronchopulmonary segment. A systemic abnormality is more likely when infection recurs in shifting sites. Recurrent pneumonia may also be caused by repeated aspiration.

Atypical pneumonia

Atypical pneumonia is a term used to describe pneumonia caused by organisms other than the classical bacteria. These organisms include viruses (especially influenza), coxiella, chlamydia, mycoplasma and legionella. The illness most often affects young, previously healthy people and commonly occurs in localized outbreaks.

The patient usually presents with a generalized illness, including mild to moderate fever, headache, myalgia and malaise. Thus, the patient is usually not nearly as toxic as with classical pneumonia due to pyogenic bacteria and the onset is more gradual. Respiratory symptoms are often minor, at least initially. There may be a cough but it is usually unproductive. The physical findings are often minimal but may include areas of decreased breath sounds and a few crackles. The presence of prominent non-respiratory features, particularly involving the brain, gut or kidney, should suggest the possibility of Legionnaires' disease. Although atypical pneumonia is usually relatively mild, it can at times be severe and even fatal (especially legionella and influenzal pneumonia).

The chest X-ray changes are generally much greater than the physical findings would suggest. Haematological examination shows a mild to moderate leucocytosis, usually with a lymphocytosis. Microbiological examination of sputum is usually unrewarding and the aetiological agent is most readily identified from serial serology, although it may be obtained from direct immunofluorescence or special culture. Arterial blood gas analysis is required if respiratory failure is suspected.

The treatment should comprise erythromycin (0.5−1 g 6 hourly) or doxycycline (100 mg 12 hourly) because atypical organisms, except viruses, are sensitive to these antibiotics. Treatment should continue for up to 3 weeks. The occasional severe case will also need supportive treatment for respiratory failure.

Hospital-acquired pneumonia

Hospital-acquired or nosocomial pneumonia has become a major cause of morbidity and mortality in hospital patients, particularly the increasing population of patients who are old or frail, have major underlying disease, have been subjected to invasive respiratory therapy, or have recent surgical wounds or infected foci elsewhere (especially of the gastrointestinal or renal tracts). The organisms involved in hospital-acquired pneumonia are quite different from those causing community-acquired pneumonia. The latter is usually pneumococcal or viral; in milder cases, mycoplasma may be involved and in more severe cases, staphylococci (especially after influenza) and Gram-negative bacilli (especially in alcoholics). Many cases of community-acquired pneumonia are not severe enough to be hospitalized.

By contrast, in hospital-acquired pneumonia, the infective organisms are usually aerobic Gram-negative bacilli and sometimes staphylococci. Many of these organisms are multi-antibiotic resistant. The aerobic Gram-negative organisms include chiefly *E. coli*. klebsiella, proteus and pseudomonas. Anaerobes are particularly seen in patients who have impaired consciousness and are at risk from aspiration of contaminated oropharyngeal secretions into the lower respiratory tract. The organisms involved are usually mixed and include bacteroides and oral anaerobes, either alone or in combination with more classical aerobic organisms.

Clinical and radiological findings are those of broncho-pneumonia superimposed on an underlying respiratory or other disorder. Such pneumonias span the whole spectrum from relatively mild and indolent processes to life-threatening infections associated with septicaemia, respiratory failure and shock. Abscess formation is prominent with pseudomonal, staphylococcal and mixed anaerobic infections, the latter frequently giving rise to a severe necrotizing pneumonia with putrid sputum. The choice of antibiotics should be guided particularly by the known sensitivity patterns of the likely organisms in the particular institution. In general, the Gram-negative infections will require an aminoglycoside (gentamicin, tobramycin, amikacin) and/or a new penicillin (ticarcillin, piperacillin, mezlocillin) or a later cephalosporin (e.g. cefotaxime, ceftazidime) or one of a number of new groups of antibiotics (e.g. imipenem, aztreonam). Staphylococci may be resistant to all antibiotics except vancomycin. Anaerobic infections require metronidazole or clindamycin.

Pneumonia in the compromised host

Although most of the patients who develop hospital-acquired pneumonia are compromised hosts in one way or another, the term is more commonly used to refer to those patients, in hospital or not, who have specific impairment of their host defences. These conditions include immune diseases (e.g. the acquired immune deficiency syndrome), haematological or other malignancies, immunosuppressive, cytotoxic or corticosteroid therapy, organ transplantation, diabetes, uraemia and sarcoidosis.

While pneumonia in such patients is commonly caused by the usual primary pathogens, infection from opportunistic organisms of relatively low virulence also occurs. These latter organisms include viruses (especially cytomegalovirus and herpes simplex virus), Gram-negative bacteria, fungi (especially *Candida sp.*) and protozoa (especially *Pneumocystis carinii*). Immune deficiencies involving IgG, neutrophils or complement are particularly associated with bacterial infection, whereas T cell deficiency is more usually associated with viral, fungal or protozoal infection.

The clinical findings are similar to those of pneumonia in other situations, except that a prominent underlying disease is also present. The pneumonia is often severe, with acute respiratory failure requiring major supportive therapy. The specific diagnosis, however, is often difficult and a sick compromised host with a pulmonary infiltrate frequently presents a considerable diagnostic problem. More complex diagnostic methods have often to be employed, especially fibreoptic bronchoscopy with washings, lavage and sometimes transbronchial lung biopsy.

Specific diagnosis is important because many opportunistic infections have effective specific treatment. This includes acyclovir for herpes simplex virus, aminoglycosides and new pencillins for Gram-negative organisms, amphotericin for candida, and cotrimoxazole for pneumocystis.

Exotic pneumonia

Exotic pneumonia is the term applied to infection due to an unusual organism. This organism may be either common, though not as a respiratory pathogen, or else uncommon and infectious by virtue of an unusual environment.

● The *common organisms* include some viruses and coxiellae, bacteria such as atypical mycobacteria and actinomyces, fungi such as aspergillus and cryptococcus, and some protozoa. These organisms cause pneumonia mainly in compromised hosts and in these patients the diagnostic net has to be cast somewhat wider than usual if one of the more expected organisms is not readily isolated.

● The *uncommon organisms* include bacteria giving rise to melioidosis, nocardiosis, plague, anthrax and tularaemia, and many fungi which have restricted geographical distribution, such as histoplasma, coccidioimyces and blastomyces. These organisms are generally identifiable, provided there is a high level of clinical suspicion of unusual pathogens in patients who may have acquired their infection in an unfamiliar environment, usually as travellers.

Necrotizing pneumonia, lung abscess, empyema

Necrotizing pneumonia, lung abscess and empyema represent the extreme of pyogenic infection in the lung. Fortunately, they have become much less common than in former years. Necrotizing pneumonia leading to abscess formation is typically caused by klebsiella, staphylococci, pseudomonas and mixed anaerobic infections. Necrotic infective cavities also occur in tuberculosis, fungal infections, carcinoma, infected cysts, septic infarcts and diffuse vasculitis. The diagnosis is made radiologically and the causative organisms identified by sputum examination. The prognosis nowadays is generally good, since the responsible infection is likely to respond well to antibiotics though the course may need to be prolonged. Surgical resection is rarely needed.

Empyema refers to a purulent pleural effusion. The usual cause is extension from adjacent pneumonia or abscess (lung, subphrenic). The organisms involved are those of the original infection. Empyema is an important complication and one of the causes of failure of resolution of infection. The clinical features are those of persistent infection together with the signs of pleural effusion and, if diagnosis is delayed, finger clubbing. Diagnosis is established by chest X-ray and needle aspiration of pus. Treatment consists of prolonged antibiotic therapy and drainage. Decortication of organized, thickened pleura is occasionally required.

Tuberculosis

Tuberculosis has been one of the major epidemics of mankind since before recorded history. Although its prevalence and mortality have progressively declined over the past century to very low levels in developed countries, it remains a major problem in developing countries. Even in developed countries, tuberculosis still occurs with sufficient frequency for clinical suspicion to remain high, especially in population sub-groups, such as indigenous, migrant, deprived or institutionalized people. The mortality from tuberculosis is now about one per 100 000 population in developed countries and its incidence about 15 per 100 000 population per year.

As is well known, the disease is caused by the organism *Mycobacterium tuberculosis*, an acid-fast aerobic bacillus of considerable robustness and longevity. Its acquisition is virtually always by inhalation. The initial, 'primary' infection consists of a small focus of peripheral consolidation with associated lymphadenopathy. Hypersensitivity of the cell-mediated type then occurs and the primary complex usually heals completely, often with calcification, but dormant organisms may remain. Occasionally, the primary infection may lead to haematogenous spread with disseminated or miliary tuberculosis or tuberculous meningitis.

The occurrence of later, pulmonary tuberculosis ('post-primary' or 'adult' tuberculosis) is usually due to reactivation, though it may be due to reinfection. This form of tuberculosis is the most frequent type clinically encountered and is the main source of infection for others. The lesion is usually in the upper zone of the lung and consists of necrosis and cavitation with chiefly bronchial spread.

The clinical features of tuberculosis are very variable. Sometimes the patient is asymptomatic and is detected at incidental radiological examination. Systemic symptoms, however, are usual, with fever, night sweats, malaise and weight loss. Respiratory symptoms are dominated by cough. There may be variable sputum, haemoptysis, chest pain, dyspnoea or wheeze. There may be recurrent colds or poorly resolving pneumonia. There is frequently an underlying condition, such as diabetes, corticosteroid therapy, alcoholism or recent upper gastrointestinal surgery. Physical examination typically shows fever, tachycardia and occasionally clubbing. Examination of the chest may be normal or may show variable findings of upper zone crackles, consolidation, pleural effusion or rarely cavitation. Cor pulmonale is present in advanced disease. Chest X-ray is always abnormal and may show upper zone shadows, cavitation, calcification, fibrosis and tracheal deviation. However, these changes though characteristic are not specific for tuberculosis. Chronicity on serial examination is typical.

Sputum examination includes direct smear as well as culture, the latter taking up to 6 weeks. False positive results are rare but false negative results are not uncommon. The Mantoux test is virtually always positive except in the presence of anergy. Biopsy of pleura, lymph node, liver or bone marrow may reveal the presence of caseating granulomas and may be culture-positive. Lung function is disturbed to a varying degree and tests may show restriction and reduced lung volumes, obstruction, decreased gas transfer and pulmonary hypertension in more advanced disease.

Definitive diagnosis requires the demonstration of the responsible organism and the presence of an appropriate lesion. The differential diagnosis includes, among others, the different causes of diffuse lung shadowing, lung nodules, cavitation or pleural effusion (see Chapter 21).

Complications include pleurisy and pleural effusion, tuberculosis in extrapulmonary sites (such as lymph nodes, urogenital system, bones, joints, pericardium and peritoneum) and hypokalaemia.

Treatment is in recent times so effective that if it could be reliably applied in all causes, the disease would likely disappear. This has not been possible for logistic and economic rather than scientific reasons. Combination chemotherapy of two or three drugs has been the mainstay of treatment for over 30 years. The efficacy of current regimens using first-line drugs under careful supervision has permitted the duration of therapy to be reduced from 18 or more months to 6 or 9 months (i.e. 'short-course') in most cases. Antibiotic sensitivity to the various antituberculous drugs should be demonstrated microbiologically. Primary drug resistance is not common but is increasing and is encouraged by poor drug compliance. Isoniazid (300 mg) and rifampicin (600 mg) is a popular combination given as a single daily dose. Streptomycin may be added for cavitary lesions and pyrazinamide for closed lesions. Otherwise, streptomycin is not now commonly used, except in developing countries where the cost of rifampicin is a problem. Second-line drugs include ethambutol, para-aminosalicylic acid (PAS), ethionamide, cycloserine and thiacetazone.

The chief side-effects of the main antituberculous drugs are shown in Table 12.3. Since large numbers of patients are treated

Isoniazid
  hepatitis, peripheral neuritis
Rifampicin
  hepatitis, fever, purpura,
  decreased effectiveness of contraceptive pill
  and oral anticoagulants
Streptomycin
  vestibular damage, ototoxicity
Pyrazinamide
  hepatitis
Ethambutol
  optic neuritis
Para-aminosalicylic acid
  gastrointestinal disturbance, fever
Ethionamide
  hepatitis,
  gastrointestinal disturbance

for prolonged periods with multiple drugs, such side-effects become of considerable importance, especially as their occurrence is relatively frequent and their nature potentially severe. Corticosteroids are of value in the inital treatment of seriously ill patients. Isolation is necessary only while the patient has positive sputum. Important aspects of tuberculosis control include surveying of the close contacts of new cases and the long-term follow-up of treated cases.

Prophylaxis is a complex issue but, in general, vaccination with BCG is indicated in communities with a significant prevalence rate or in inidividuals in high-risk groups, and chemoprophylaxis with isoniazid for 6 months is indicated in exposed individuals with positive Mantoux tests. Tuberculosis control overall is a public health task of considerable complexity and magnitude.

Pulmonary disease due to non-tuberculous mycobacteria

Mycobacteria of many species are widely distributed in the environment. The finding of resistant mycobacteria, in some cases diagnosed as tuberculosis, led to the realization that other mycobacteria previously thought saprophytic could at times be pathogenic, and to the subsequent taxonomic clarification of the many species involved. Two of these, *M. avium-intracellulare* and *M. kansasii*, have been clearly implicated in clinical pulmonary disease. The source of infection is usually the environment rather than another person. The manifestations are very similar to those of classical tuberculosis. Atypical mycobacteria may also cause cervical lymphadenitis. Pulmonary disease due to these organisms tends to be both more indolent and more resistant to therapy. Multiple drug regimens are required, based on sensitivity testing.

Sarcoidosis	Angiitis and granulomatosis
Diffuse fibrosing alveolitis	Wegener's granulomatosis
Histiocytosis X	Lymphomatoid
Haemorrhagic infiltrates	granulomatosis
Goodpasture's syndrome	Bronchocentric
Idiopathic pulmonary	granulomatosis
haemosiderosis	Rare pulmonary infiltrative
Pulmonary infiltration with	conditions
eosinophilia (PIE)	Pulmonary alveolar
Loeffler's syndrome	proteinosis
Asthmatic pulmonary eosinophilia	Pulmonary alveolar
Tropical pulmonary eosinophilia	microlithiasis
Eosinophilic pneumonia	Lymphangiomyomatosis
	Pulmonary amyloidosis

The interstitial lung diseases are a group of diffuse pulmonary processes, many of unknown aetiology. Specific interstitial diseases such as pneumonia, pulmonary oedema, pneumo-conioses and other occupational lung diseases, drug reactions and lung involvement in systemic diseases are considered elsewhere.

Sarcoidosis

Although sarcoidosis is a systemic disease, its chief manifestations are pulmonary. It is a relatively common condition of unknown aetiology. Since there are no individual or collective pathognomonic features, clinical investigations or histology, an international conference prepared the following description to serve in place of a definition for the time being (see Hinshaw & Murray, 1980 and Crofton & Douglas, 1981).

'Sarcoidosis is a multisystem granulomatous disorder of unknown aetiology most commonly affecting young adults and presenting most frequently with bilateral hilar lymphadeno-pathy, pulmonary infiltration, skin or eye lesions. The diagnosis is established most securely when clinicoradiographic findings are supported by histological evidence of widespread non-caseating epithelioid-cell granulomas in more than one organ or by a positive Kveim−Siltzbach skin test. Immunological features are depression of delayed-type hypersensitivity suggesting impaired cell-mediated immunity and raised or abnormal immunoglobulins. There may be hypercalciuria, with or without hypercalcaemia. The course and prognosis may correlate with mode of onset: an acute onset with erythema nodosum heralds a self-limiting course and spontaneous resolution, whereas an insidious onset may be followed by relentless progressive fibrosis. Corticosteroids relieve symptoms and suppress inflammation and granuloma formation'.

Sarcoidosis occurs mainly in young adults. It is also more common in temperate than in tropical climates. The incidence mostly ranges from 5−20 per 100 000 population.

The aetiology is most likely to be one or more, as yet unidentified, transmittable agents. The possibility of an atypical reaction to tuberculosis or other mycobacterium (or other known organism) is not nowadays considered tenable. There appears to be some genetic predisposition. There is depressed cell-mediated immunity (anergy) but often enhanced humoral or B lymphocyte activity.

The clinical features of sarcoidosis are so protean that it has been pointed out that patients may present not only to a chest physician but also to the cardiologist, dermatologist, gastro-enterologist, neurologist, ophthalmologist or rheumatologist as well as to a general physician or surgeon. In fact, pulmonary involvement occurs in about 90% of cases. It is classified on the basis of the chest X-ray as:

- *Stage I* with bilateral hilar adenopathy (50% of cases).
- *Stage II* with bilateral hilar adenopathy plus pulmonary infiltration (25% of cases).
- *Stage III* with pulmonary infiltration only (15% of cases).

The remaining 10% of cases have normal chest X-rays and are sometimes referred to as *Stage O*. There is no necessary progression or retrogression serially through the individual stages.

Pulmonary involvement is the major cause of disability and death in sarcoidosis. Dyspnoea is common and may occur even in Stage I. Dry cough and chest discomfort may occur as well as systemic symptoms such as fatigue, malaise and weight loss. Erythema nodosum and arthralgia are common presenting complaints in patients without respiratory symptoms who have Stage I disease. Symptoms correlate much better with functional or pathological changes than with radiological changes, the latter often being either considerably greater or less than the symptoms would suggest. Physical examination of the chest is frequently normal but crackles and rhonchi are sometimes noted. Extrapulmonary manifestations are numerous and varied (Tabel 13.1).

Diffuse pulmonary involvement may be miliary, nodular or reticular. Confluent infiltrates may occur and are sometimes massive. The respiratory tract may also be affected in other

Table 13.1. Extrapulmonary manifestations of sarcoidosis

Lymphadenopathy
Uveitis, keratoconjunctivitis sicca, retinopathy
Salivary gland enlargement, fever
Erythema nodosum, skin nodules, maculopapular rash, lupus pernio
Hepatomegaly, splenomegaly
Bone cysts, polyarthralgia, myopathy
Peripheral neuropathy, meningitis, intracranial space-occupying lesions, hypothalamic involvement
Disordered calcium metabolism, hypercalcaemia, hypercalciuria, nephrocalcinosis
Myocardial granulomas

ways such as with nasal granuloma, laryngeal plaques and pleural effusion. An unusual variant is necrotizing sarcoid granulomatosis with pulmonary arteritis.

Chest radiography is always essential as clinically silent pulmonary involvement is usual, even if the presentation is extrapulmonary. Lung function tests may show decreased ventilatory capacity (usually restrictive but occasionally obstructive in pattern), hypoxaemia and hypocapnia, decreased lung volumes, decreased compliance and decreased gas transfer. The latter is probably the most sensitive functional test and the best for serial follow-up. Although these functional changes correlate quite well with pathological changes, they are not helpful prognostically. The Mantoux test is negative and the Kveim test postive in about 80% of cases. Microbiological examination of sputum should exclude acid-fast bacilli. Hypercalcaemia and hypercalciuria may occur. The serum angiotensin converting enzyme (ACE) level is increased in most acute patients and a gallium scan often shows abnormal pulmonary uptake. Biopsy of lymph node, Kveim nodule, lung or other tissue and histological demonstration of non-caseating granulomas are usually essential for diagnosis.

Treatment is not required in many patients because the disability is mild and remission is usual. Corticosteroids can suppress the manifestations of acute sarcoidosis but whether they alter the long-term outcome remains unproven. Most clinicians, however, would use a prolonged course of corticosteroids in Stage II or III disease with dyspnoea and abnormal lung function and in serious extrapulmonary disease.

The prognosis is usually good because about 80% of patients with Stage I disease undergo a complete remission within 1 to 2 years. In about 10% of patients, progression to fibrosis occurs. Severe chronic extrapulmonary lesions are usually associated with pulmonary fibrosis. The overall mortality is less than 5% and is most commonly due to respiratory failure secondary to severe pulmonary fibrosis.

Diffuse fibrosing alveolitis (interstitial pneumonitis, idiopathic pulmonary fibrosis, cryptogenic fibrosing alveolitis, Hamman–Rich syndrome)

This is a form of progressive diffuse inflammation, distal to the terminal bronchiole. Although its aetiology is unknown and no single pathogenetic mechanism has yet been defined, there are common histological, radiological and clinical features exhibited by most patients with this condition, justifying its consideration as a separate entity. However, it may well represent a group of disorders and in any event is not easy to distinguish from similar processes associated with systemic disease or certain drugs.

Aetiological factors may well be immunological because, although no specific antigen has been identifiable, both cell-mediated and humoral changes can be shown and circulating immune complexes demonstrated in the cellular, pre-fibrotic stage of disease. An association with other auto-immune diseases has sometimes been found and there appears to be some genetic predisposition. No infective agent has yet been identified.

The pathological changes consist of:

1 Thickening of alveolar walls due to inflammatory cells, leading to fibrosis.

2 The presence within the alveoli of large mononuclear cells, mainly desquamated type 2 pneumocytes but also macrophages.

A better corticosteroid response is likely to occur when the latter changes are more prominent and the former changes less prominent. Eventually, cellularity decreases and fibrosis increases, so that the alveolar architecture is completely disorganized with fibrosis and the appearance of cystic spaces (honeycombing). These processes, though diffuse, are not uniform throughout the lung.

The clinical features are usually dominated by progressive dyspnoea. The first presentation is sometimes as an apparent acute respiratory infection. A dry cough is common, as is fever and weight loss. On physical examination, there is frequently cyanosis, clubbing and tachypnoea. Diffuse crackles are heard, particularly at the lung bases. A late finding is cor pulmonale. Even in the absence of a definable systemic disease, extrapulmonary manifestations may occur, such as Raynaud's phenomenon and hyponatraemia.

The chest X-ray may initially be normal, even in the presence of dyspnoea. The radiological abnormalities tend to be diffuse, homogeneous or nodular opacities at first, reticulonodular later and eventually reticular, often with honeycombing. Lung function tests show changes similar to those described for sarcoidosis. Lung biopsy is required for definitive diagnosis, though a clinical diagnosis may sometimes be relied upon if the patient is particularly unwell or the features are unequivocal. A common controversy surrounds the need for lung biopsy, especially open biopsy, when the histological result will be non-specific and no major therapeutic option other than corticosteroids is available. A more scientific view would support the desirability for maximum knowledge in at least most cases, provided it can be obtained with reasonable cost and safety.

Treatment is virtually confined to corticosteroids. In some patients, there is a dramatic response but in most there is continued progression, despite some symptomatic amelioration. Treatment is long-term and dosage should be titrated not only against symptoms but also appropriate lung function tests, particularly those of gas exchange. The place of immunosuppressive and anti-inflammatory therapy is unresolved. Complications such as supervening infection and heart failure should be treated on their merits. Long-term oxygen therapy may be symptomatically helpful.

The course of the disease is very variable. The mean time from onset of symptoms to death is 3 to 4 years though reported survival has ranged from 1 month to over 20 years. The duration of survival appears to correlate with the severity of disease at the time of diagnosis and the prognosis is better in patients with acute desquamative forms of disease with little fibrosis. In fact, desquamative interstitial pneumonitis is regarded as a separate entity by some. Occasionally, spontaneous or corticosteroid-induced remissions occur.

Histiocytosis X

Histiocytosis X comprises three related diseases — eosinophilic granuloma, Hand—Schuller—Christian disease and Letterer—Siwe disease. All consist of granulomatous infiltration with large histiocytes containing foamy eosinophilic cytoplasm.
- *Eosiophilic granuloma* is seen only in adults. It is relatively benign, frequently asymptomatic and often remits. The patient usually presents with an unexpected diffuse pulmonary infiltrate or sometimes an osteolytic bone lesion. In some patients, interstitial fibrosis may develop with honeycombing and a tendency to pneumothorax.
- *Hand—Schuller—Christian disease* occurs in children as well as adults. It is a multi-system disease affecting bone particularly. Diabetes insipidus is common. Pulmonary involvement may include progressive fibrosis with honeycombing.
- *Letterer—Siwe disease* occurs only in infants.

The diagnosis of histiocytosis X requires histological confirmation. Treatment of symptomatic patients is with corticosteroids and perhaps immunosuppressive thereapy.

Haemorrhagic infiltrates

Goodpasture's syndrome

This comprises interstitial and alveolar haemorrhage with haemoptysis, anaemia and glomerulonephritis. It is an autoimmune disease, associated with antiglomerular (and alveolar) basement membrane antibodies. It is generally a disease of young adult males. There is a patchy, variable pulmonary infiltrate, initially due to haemorrhage and later fibrosis. Diagnosis is based on renal or lung biopsy and the demonstration of circulating antiglomerular basement membrane antibodies. Until recently, the mortality was very high despite corticosteroids, immunosuppressive therapy and even bilateral nephrectomy. Nowadays, plasmapheresis is the treatment of choice and the outcome is dramatically improved.

Idiopathic pulmonary haemosiderosis

This is a rare disease indistinguishable from the pulmonary component of Goodpasture's syndrome and occurring mainly in children. It is often fatal, although the prognosis appears very variable and there is no clearly effective therapy.

Pulmonary infiltration with eosinophilia (PIE)

This group of conditions includes Loeffler's syndrome, asthmatic pulmonary eosinophilia, tropical eosinophilia and eosinophilic pneumonia. Specific conditions such as eosinophilic leukaemia, polyarteritis nodosa, Hodgkin's disease and hydatid disease may also give rise to pulmonary infiltration in association with blood eosinophilia.

Loeffler's syndrome

Otherwise known as simple pulmonary eosinophilia, this consists of transient and variable pulmonary infiltrates, associated with a high white cell count (up to 20 x 10^9/l) and eosinophil count (up to 20% or more). It generally lasts less than a month but may occasionally last up to 6 months or more. It is probably due to an allergic reaction to a variety of possible allergens, particularly helminths. Most cases are clinically silent but cough and systemic symptoms sometimes occur. Recovery is invariable and treatment is not indicated.

Asthmatic pulmonary eosinophilia

This is characterized by asthma with recurrent, variable and changing shadows on chest X-ray and variable eosinophilia. Most cases are associated with *Aspergillus fumigatus* colonization and the fungus acts as an antigen. Typically, the patient is febrile during acute exacerbations and coughs up brown plugs or bronchial casts containing eosinophils and fungal mycelia. Mucoid impaction may occur with bronchial obstruction due to inspissated mucus. Bronchiectasis and lobar shrinkage may be found. Precipitins for *Aspergillus fumigatus* are usually present in serum. The course is generally chronic and treatment is as for asthma, with corticosteroids usually required. Specific antifungal therapy is unhelpful.

Tropical pulmonary eosinophilia

This is now known to be an allergic reaction to filaria. The patient presents with episodic fever, cough, wheeze and often systemic symptoms. Untreated, alternating recurrences and remissions may persist for years. Treatment is with diethylcarbamazine.

Eosinophilic pneumonia

This is a syndrome of fever, weight loss, dyspnoea, wheeze, very marked eosinophilia and peripheral infiltrates on chest X-ray, associated with histological changes similar to those of other PIE conditions. These features are non-specific but in toto characteristic. Its aetiology is unknown and diagnosis usually requires lung biopsy. The condition responds dramatically to corticosteroids.

Angiitis and granulomatosis

Wegener's granulomatosis

This consists of a necrotizing granulomatous vasculitis of the upper (nose, sinuses) and lower respiratory tract and kidneys. A limited form may affect the lungs only. The aetiology is unknown but the pathogenesis appears immunological and may involve the production of immune complexes and thus of aggressive, malignant granulomas or vasculitis. The patient typically presents with cough, pleuritic pain and haemoptysis. There may be symptoms of multi-organ involvement. The chest X-ray shows single or multiple densities of varying size, often with cavitation, or sometimes a more general infiltration. The condition is often initially misdiagnosed as pulmonary malignancy, but histolgical examination establishes the diagnosis. The course of illness was rapidly fatal until the advent of corticosteroids and cytotoxic therapy. Long-term remission is now usual.

Lymphomatoid granulomatosis

An uncommon condition, this has histological features resembling both Wegener's granulomatosis and lymphoma.

There is a pulmonary infiltrate which is angiocentric, destructive and lymphoreticular, with atypical cells showing mitoses. Similar lesions may be found in other organs, especially skin and sometimes the mouth. Respiratory symptoms include cough, sputum and dyspnoea. The chest X-ray shows bilateral infiltrates, rounded lesions similar to metastases and cavitation. There is a high mortality, often with progression to malignant lymphoma. No consistently effective treatment is available, although corticosteroids are generally used and recent reports of combined corticosteroid and cytotoxic therapy are promising.

Bronchocentric granulomatosis

This is a destructive condition similar to Wegener's granulomatosis, except that the lesions are centred on bronchi and not on blood vessels. The distinction is important because its prognosis is much better. Many patients have asthma, eosinophilia, mucus plugs and hypersensitivity to *Aspergillus fumigatus*, and in these it may represent a variant of 'mucoid impaction'.

Rare pulmonary infiltrative conditions

Pulmonary alveolar proteinosis

This is characterized by alveolar deposition of amorphous, eosinophilic, PAS-positive proteinaceous material. This material contains lipid and glycoprotein and bears some resemblance to surfactant. The lung structure is undisturbed. Its aetiology and pathogenesis are unknown but it may represent defective clearance of surfactant. Clinical features vary from no significant disability to those of respiratory failure, largely depending on the extent of involvement. Secondary infection may occur, especially with fungi. The chest X-ray shows a bilateral butterfly-shaped infiltrate. Many patients have a spontaneous remission and only a few are seriously ill. There is no specific therapy and in particular, corticosteroids are contraindicated, but lung lavage is useful if symptoms are marked.

Pulmonary alveolar microlithiasis

A rare and mysterious condition, this is characterized by intra-alveolar deposition of calcium-laden concretions which appear as diffuse, tiny, dense particles on chest X-ray. There is no known treatment and most patients are asymptomatic.

Lymphangiomyomatosis

This is a progressive, diffuse, interstitial process characterized by smooth muscle proliferation in lung and lymphatic tissue. It occurs in younger women and may be associated with a chylous pleural effusion. The prognosis is poor in advanced disease and there appears to be no effective therapy.

Pulmonary amyloidosis

This may rarely occur as either a primary (submucosal and thus obstructive) or secondary (infiltrative) condition.

Aspiration pneumonitis
Drowning
Pulmonary reactions to drugs and
  poisons
Occupational lung diseases
  Pneumoconiosis
  Occupational asthma
  Hypersensitivity pneumonitis
  Acute lung irritation
  Occupational pulmonary
    infections

Occupational lung diseases *cont.*
  Occupational pulmonary
    neoplasms
  Miscellaneous occupational
    lung diseases
Trauma
Burns
Radiation

Aspiration pneumonitis (chemical pneumonia, Mendelson's syndrome)

Aspiration pneumonitis refers to the inhalation of gastric contents. The aspiration of upper respiratory tract material as a cause of pneumonia has already been referred to (see Chapter 12). Aspiration of gastric contents is a serious complication in patients with airways unprotected because of impaired consciousness and/or disturbance of gastro-oesophageal function. The original description of this condition was in obstetrical patients, in whom it is still a significant problem. Many of the procedures in caring for the unconscious patient, particularly in anaesthesia, relate to airway protection and thus prevention of aspiration.

The pathogenesis is related to the acidity of the gastric contents and damage is especially significant when the pH is less than 2.5. Acid inhalation causes immediate chemical damage to the bronchial mucosal cells or alveolar epithelial cells, with resulting inflammatory exudate and cellular infiltrate.

The clinical features start with the aspiration event itself, which may be observed. Immediate asphyxia may occasionally result, especially if the aspiration is large and particulate. More typically, cough, frothy sputum, dyspnoea and wheeze occur, usually within an hour or so. The features of bronchopneumonia become apparent within 24–48 hours. Secondary aerobic or anaerobic infection may occur in the next few days. Hypoxaemia is sometimes severe. Specific problems occur if the aspiration is infected or if large food particles are retained. Hydrocarbon pneumonitis may result from the aspiration of kerosene, petrol, polish, solvent and some insecticides. If the aspirate includes mineral oil, formerly a popular nighttime laxative, *chronic lipoid pneumonia* can be produced by repeated aspiration.

The diagnosis is often straightforward but may be difficult if the aspiration has not been witnessed, if the patient is already ill for other reasons or if no food particles or patchy inflammation are found in the tracheobronchial tree at bronchoscopy. Conversely, if food particles are found in the oropharynx, a mistaken diagnosis of aspiration may be made in other situations.

The treatment is supportive. Since the chemical reaction is immediate, measures such as instillation of bicarbonate or saline lavage are not helpful. Corticosteroids have been shown to be ineffective and prophylactic antibiotics are generally contraindicated. Treatment consists of oxygenation, cardiovascular resuscitation if necessary, intubation and mechanical ventilation in seriously affected patients, and bronchodilators when bronchospasm is prominent.

Drowning

Drowning and near-drowning are common accidents in most societies. Differences used to be claimed between drowning in salt water and in fresh water. Aspiration of hypertonic salt water (5% saline) was though to cause haemoconcentration, whereas aspiration of hypotonic fresh water was thought to cause haemodilution, haemolysis and hyperkalaemia. In fact, intense reflex laryngospasm with resultant asphyxia is the usual cause of death and water enters the lungs mainly as a terminal event. Pathological changes after drowning and clinical and investigational findings after near-drowning are similar for both sea or fresh water.

Patients rescued after near-drowning are comatose and apnoeic. Even after resuscitation, central nervous system changes including confusion, restlessness, delirium and convulsions may persist for a variable time. Hypothermia is frequently followed by mild fever. Respiratory features include tachypnoea, cough, frothy blood-stained sputum, chest pain and wheeze. Respiratory failure may occur some hours later. Circulatory changes include tachycardia, arrhythmias and sometimes hypertension. Gastric distension and vomiting may occur.

Investigations show arterial hypoxaemia, variable serum electrolyte levels and albuminuria, haematuria and occasionally haemoglobinuria. The chest X-ray usually shows perihilar densities initially, although it may be normal, and more florid pulmonary oedema is common some hours later.

Treatment consists of urgent cardiopulmonary resuscitation and subsequent oxygenation, endotracheal intubation and mechanical ventilation if necessary. Nasogastric aspiration is advisable. The use of corticosteroids is of unproven value and prophylactic antibiotics are contraindicated.

Pulmonary reactions to drugs and poisons

A number of different pulmonary reactions involving a large variety of drugs and poisons may occur. Although they are less common than drug-induced reactions involving other organs and systems, they are important because they can be severe and life-threatening, they are often reversible if the responsible drug is ceased and they can mimic other more common respiratory diseases. The mechanisms of drug-induced reactions are probably many and among others include immunological (allergic) and pharmacological (idiosyncratic, facilitative, toxic) processes.

The different clinical presentations of pulmonary reactions are listed in Table 14.1 together with the drugs and other agents most frequently involved.

Table 14.1. Pulmonary reactions to drugs and other agents

Bronchospasm	
Type 1 hypersensitivity	antibiotics (especially penicillin)
	antisera
	iodides (especially contrast media)
	iron-dextran
Irritant reflexes	acetylcysteine
	aerosols (especially cromoglycate)
	ß-adrenergic blockers
Smooth muscle contraction	**histamine**
	methacholine
	PGF$_2\alpha$
Prostaglandin inhibition	**aspirin**
	other NSAIDs
Interstitial infiltration	
Acute (usually with eosinophilia)	azathioprine
	gold
	isoniazid
	nitrofurantoin
	PAS
	penicillin
	sulphonamides
	tricyclic antidepressants
Chronic	**bleomycin**
	busulfan
	cyclophosphamide
	gold
	hexamethonium
	melphalan
	methysergide
	nitrofurantoin
	oxygen
SLE-like	digitalis
	gold
	griseofulvin
	hydrallazine
	isoniazid
	methyldopa
	oral contraceptives
	penicillin
	phenytoin
	procainamide
	reserpine
	sulphonamides
	tetracyclines
	thiazides
Pulmonary oedema	
Increased hydrostatic pressure	adrenaline
	i.v. fluids
	propranolol
Increased capillary permeability	blood transfusion
	dextropropoxyphene
	heroin
	salicylates
	thiazides

122/*Chapter 14*

Table 14.1. *contd*

Pulmonary vascular changes	
Pulmonary hypertension	aminorex
	talc
Vasculitis	hydrallazine
	penicillin
	phenytoin
	promazine
	quinidine
	sulphonamides
Respiratory failure	
CNS depression	alchohol
	anaesthetics
	opiates
	sedatives
Neuromuscular blockade	aminoglycosides
	muscle relaxants
Pulmonary haemorrhage	anticoagulants
	antiplatelet agents
	thrombolytic agents
Hilar lymphadenopathy	phenytoin

Drugs printed in bold type are those most frequently involved in the particular reaction. NSAID = non-steroidal anti-inflammatory drug; CNS = central nervous system.

The diagnosis of a drug-induced pulmonary reaction is usually presumptive. Clinical suspicion is complemented by a careful history rather than laboratory tests. Even in allergic reactions, serum antibody levels and skin tests are not usually helpful. The suspected offending drug should be stopped and most reactions then subside, though some pulmonary infiltrates may take weeks to resolve. Corticosteroid therapy may hasten the resolution of infiltrative reactions but other reactions should be treated on their symptomatic merits. Rechallenge with the responsible drug would be diagnostically confirmatory but is usually unsafe. Many reactions are such that the patient should be warned about possible future exposure to the drug.

Occupational lung diseases Lung damage from inhalation of dusts, fumes or other injurious substances may occur in certain occupations in most societies, especially the industrialized. There is a vast number of such substances and the consequences of their inhalation range from minor to severe. Fortunately, most substances to which the population is exposed are not harmful and those that are injurious are probably well recognized nowadays, so that appropriate preventive measures can be taken. The occupational lung diseases may be classified into the pneumoconioses, occupational asthma, hypersensitivity pneumonitis, acute lung irritation, occupational infections, malignancy and a large and heterogeneous group of miscellaneous diseases.

Pneumoconiosis

This refers to the permanent accumulation of inhaled dust in the lungs together with the tissue reaction to its presence. Pneumoconiosis is thus not a single disease but a process common to a number of different specific entities. A dust is an aerosol of solid, inanimate particles whose size needs to be less than 10 μm to be retained in the lung. This size is somewhat unusual, especially in nature, and requires the disruptive forces of industrial processes. Moreover, only a few specific dusts among the many produced give rise to clinical disease and these must be inhaled in sufficient amount for a sufficient time. Finally, associated damage due to smoking is very common and may outweigh any effect of inhaled dust.

The chief pneumoconioses are due to coal dust, silica and asbestos. Coal dust and silica give rise to simple pneumoconiosis with a few or no symptoms or lung function abnormalities, but the chest X-ray shows diffuse, multiple, rounded opacities. If the silica is inhaled as very fine particles, a diffuse interstitial fibrosis rather than a nodular pathology may result. For reasons that are unclear but may be immunological, some patients develop complicated pneumoconiosis in the form of *progressive massive fibrosis* with large fibrotic lesions, often with cavities and usually in the upper lobes. Symptoms of dyspnoea and cough now appear. The progressive massive fibrosis of silicosis and of coal workers' pneumoconiosis may be complicated by tuberculosis or rheumatoid arthritis (Caplan's syndrome) respectively.

Asbestos may produce progressive, diffuse fibrosis, at which stage symptoms appear. Lung function changes, particularly decreased gas transfer, precede both symptoms and radiographic changes. In addition to producing a pneumoconiosis (asbestosis), asbestos also predisposes to calcified pleural plaques, diffuse pleural fibrosis, bronchogenic carcinoma, and pleural and peritoneal mesothelioma.

Pneumoconioses are also produced by other silicates (e.g. talc and kaolin, but not cement or fibreglass) and by aluminium, barium sulphate, iron oxide, tin oxide, tungsten carbide and beryllium, although in some of these conditions, the lung reaction is minimal. Beryllium also gives rise to diffuse granuloma formation.

Whilst radiological classification of the severity of pneumoconiosis has been attempted, in general there is a poor agreement between symptoms and functional impairment on the one hand and radiological abnormality on the other.

Occupational asthma

This may be caused by exposure to substances which are allergenic, pharmacologically active or directly irritant to the bronchial tree. Animal danders, vegetable, flower and grain dusts, wood dusts, cotton dusts, isocyanates, soldering flux, insecticides, gases (e.g. sulphur dioxide) and various chemicals and proteolytic enzymes may be incriminated. Many patients have no past history or family history of asthma and symptoms may sometimes be atypical in that wheeze is not always prominent. Typically, the symptoms are worse at work and subside at weekends and on holidays but eventually they may become chronic.

Hypersensitivity pneumonitis (extrinsic allergic alveolitis)

This is produced by the inhalation of organic dusts. There is a type III hypersensitivity reaction at the alveolar level with precipitating antibody (as opposed to the type I reaction at the bronchial level with reaginic antibody giving rise to asthma). The clinical varieties of hypersensitivity pneumonitis are listed in Table 14.2.

Unlike asthma, the clinical features of hypersensitivity pneumonitis include a marked systemic upset and the respiratory symptoms comprise cough and dyspnoea but not wheeze. On physical examination, crackles rather than rhonchi are heard and functionally there is restriction rather than obstruction. The course is usually acute, within 5−6 hours of exposure to the relevant antigen, but may be insidious. The chest X-ray shows micronodular shadows initially and fibrosis (especially of the upper lobes) later.

The diagnosis is particularly dependent on a history of appropriate exposure. Precipitating antibodies to specific antigen are detectable in acute cases but chronic disease may be difficult to distinguish from idiopathic diffuse fibrosing

Table 14.2. Types of hypersensitivity pneumonitis (extrinsic allergic alveolitis)

Conditions	Source of antigen	Precipitins present against
Bagassosis	Mouldy, overheated, sugar cane bagasse	*T. vulgaris*
Bird fancier's lung	Pigeon/budgerigar/hen/parrot proteins	Serum protein and droppings
Cheese worker's lung	Cheese mould	*Penicillium spp.*
Detergent lung	Detergents	*B. subtilis*
Farmer's lung	Mouldy hay	*M. faeni, T. vulgaris*
Humidifier fever	Forced air heating, cooling or humidification	*M. faeni*
Malt worker's lung	Mouldy barley, malt dust	*Aspergillus spp.*
Maple bark stripper's lung	Mouldy maple bark	Cryptostroma (*Coniosporium corticale*)
Mushroom worker's lung	Mushroom compost	*M. faeni, T. vulgaris*
New Guinea lung	Mouldy thatch dust	Thatch of huts
Paper-mill worker's lung	Mouldy wood pulp	*Alternaria spp.*
Paprika splitter's lung	Paprika dust	*Mucor stolonifer*
Pituitary snuff taker's lung	Heterologous pituitary powder (beef, pig)	Serum protein/pituitary antigens
Sequoiosis	Mouldy redwood sawdust	*Aureobasidium pullulans*
Suberosis	Mouldy oak bark, cork dust	*Penicillium spp.*
Wheat weevil disease	Infected wheat flour	*Sitophilus granarius*
Animal food worker's lung	Fish meal	?
Bible-printer's lung	Mouldy typesetting water	?
Blackfat tobacco smoker's lung	Blackfat tobacco	?
Coffee worker's lung	Coffee-bean extract	?
Corn farmer's lung	Corn dust	?
Furrier's lung	? Fox fur	?
Mummy-handler's lung	Mummy wrappings	?
Smallpox handler's lung	Crust from smallpox lesions	?
Tea grower's lung	Tea plants	?
Woodworker's lung	Sawdust	?

alveolitis. Lung biopsy in such patients will often shown granulomas, which then suggest the correct diagnosis. Avoidance of the offending antigen usually results in complete symptomatic remission, though some patients may remain dyspnoeic.

Acute lung irritation

This is produced by a large number of chemical atmospheric pollutants in the form of noxious gases and fumes. Irritation generally occurs in the upper respiratory tract (and often elsewhere), as well as in the lung. Clinical features thus include sneezing, rhinorrhoea, epiphora and stridor, as well as cough, wheeze and dyspnoea. Bronchiolitis, pulmonary oedema and subsequent bronchopneumonia are possible consequences. Toxic gases and fumes include ammonia, chlorine, sulphur dioxide, oxides of nitrogen, ozone, isocyanates, cadmium oxide, osmium tetroxide, metal fumes (especially oxides of zinc, copper, magnesium but also cadmium, iron, manganese, nickel, selenium, tin, antimony and vanadium), mercury, platinum salts and polymer fumes (Teflon degradation products). Systemic abnormalities are produced following the inhalation of carbon monoxide and cyanide, and asphyxia with excess carbon dioxide, nitrogen or methane.

Occupational pulmonary infections

These include tuberculosis in health workers and in miners with silicosis, Q fever in farmers, veterinarians and abattoir workers, and hydatid disease in sheep farmers.

Occupational pulmonary neoplasms

These include carcinoma of the lung associated with exposure to asbestos, uranium ore, arsenic, nickel, chromate, mustard gas and possibly other substances, and mesothelioma with asbestos.

Miscellaneous occupational lung diseases

These include:
• *Byssinosis*, found in textile workers inhaling cotton, flax or hemp dust, manifest by cough, chest tightness, dyspnoea and wheeze, especially on Mondays, with an obstructive pattern on spirometry and normal chest X-ray.
• *Thesaurosis*, a pulmonary infiltrate purportedly due to hair spray but of doubtful validity as a distinct entity.
• *Paraquat lung*, a lethal, proliferative and destructive interstitial reaction following accidental or deliberate ingestion of this toxic weed killer.

Trauma

Trauma can affect the lungs in three major ways, namely chest wall damage, pneumothorax and direct lung injury.
• *Chest wall damage* causes respiratory problems in several ways. Most obviously, when multiple ribs are fractured, there may be paradoxical movement during ventilation of that section of chest wall (flail chest). Impairment of gas exchange sufficient to require mechanical ventilation is usually due to associated pulmonary contusion rather than to the rebreathing of expired air between lung zones due to the chest wall instability (Pendelluft). However, endotracheal intubation

and mechanical ventilation are often required in severe flail chest, particularly in older patients, the indications being respiratory failure, splinting of a large flail segment or patient exhaustion.

When simple rib, costal cartilage or sternal fractures occur, there may be respiratory compromise with sputum retention because of pain and splinting, particularly in patients with lung disease. Even a simple, single rib fracture may in addition puncture the lung and cause pneumothorax.

• *Pneumothorax*, especially of the tension type, is a potentially life-threatening complication and requires urgent tube drainage to an underwater seal. It may be associated with haemothorax and there is usually accompanying subcutaneous emphysema.

• *Direct lung injury* includes pulmonary contusion or diffuse haemorrhagic damage at the site of injury. There may be a delay before radiological changes are apparent. Functional abnormalities may be severe enough to necessitate mechanical ventilation, even in the absence of flail chest. Airway disruption may sometimes occur and gives rise to mediastinal and subcutaneous emphysema and pneumothorax. Post-traumatic respiratory failure (adult respiratory distress syndrome) is a delayed complication. The possibility of associated injury of the myocardium or aorta should always be remembered in severe chest trauma.

Burns

The respiratory complications of burns can result in significant morbidity and mortality in those initially surviving a fire.

• *Direct thermal injury*, particularly of the upper respiratory tract, is common and is usually associated with facial burns. Severe acute upper airways obstruction may result. Thermal injury of the lower respiratory tract and lung parenchyma is difficult to produce except by superheated steam.

• *Smoke inhalation* is also a common thermal injury and gives rise to irritation, sometime severe, of the tracheobronchial tree. The patient may develop a chemical bronchitis, with symptoms of stridor, cough, charcoal-containing sputum, dyspnoea and wheeze. Bronchial casts may subsequently be coughed.

• *Inhalation of toxic products of combustion* results from fires in confined spaces, e.g. buildings or aircraft. These products give rise to a severe acute lung irritation syndrome, as described above in occupational lung diseases, and are a major cause of fatality.

Finally, patients with burns are at considerable risk of later respiratory complications, such as those due to pulmonary oedema (especially volume overload), adult respiratory distress syndrome and secondary bacterial infection.

Radiation

Radiation injury to the lung is an important complication of therapeutic radiation of the chest, though precautions are usually taken to minimize the exposure of normal tissues.

• *Radiation pneumonitis* is an acute, primary, vascular reaction,

127/*Other Pulmonary Insults*

initially with pulmonary vascular congestion and alveolar oedema, and later with small vessel thrombosis and alveolar epithelial desquamation. It is of variable extent and severity but occurs to some extent in all patients having chest irradiation. Symptoms appear some weeks after radiation and include dry cough and dyspnoea. The chest X-ray shows a new pulmonary infiltrate. Severe symptoms are probably helped by corticosteroids.

• *Radiation fibrosis* is a natural progression of radiation pneumonitis over the succeeding months. The chest X-ray shows infiltration and contraction of the affected part of the lung. The process is often clinically silent but dyspnoea can occur and may be progressive and disabling. There is no effective treatment.

Pulmonary Oedema

Introduction

Pulmonary oedema is defined as an increased amount of extra-vascular fluid (water and solute) in the lung. Extravascular fluid in turn may be interstitial or alveolar. Pulmonary oedema is one of the commonest respiratory disorders and may follow a wide variety of local and systemic insults. Thus, although pulmonary oedema due to left heart failure is the classical clinical picture, pulmonary oedema also occurs in a number of other common settings, such as in serious medical or surgical illness in the form of the adult respiratory distress syndrome. Pulmonary oedema can also be an important component in viral pneumonia, aspiration pneumonitis, respiratory burns, uraemia, endotoxaemia, drowning, after head injury and at altitude. In all these latter situations, the left atrial pressure may be normal or even low. Pulmonary oedema may there-fore present in diverse settings with different pathogenetic mechanisms and thus with different therapeutic implications.

Pathogenesis

The pathogenetic mechanisms of pulmonary oedema formation are still well defined by Starling's equation (1896). Thus, the net volume of fluid moving across a semi-permeable membrane is determined by the balance between the pairs of hydro-static and colloid osmotic pressures across that membrane.

Starling's equation is currently written as:

$$Jv = Kf\left[(Pc - Pt) - \sigma(\pi c - \pi t)\right]$$

where,

Jv = net volume of fluid,
Kf = capillary filtration coefficient,
Pc = capillary hydrostatic pressure,
Pt = interstitial hydrostatic pressure,
σ = capillary membrane reflection coefficient for protein,
πc = capillary oncotic pressure, and
πt = interstitial oncotic pressure.

Using average values for the lung,
$$Jv = 0.1\left[(4 - -6) - 0.8(25 - 14)\right]$$
$$= 0.1(10 - 9)$$
$$= 0.1\ \text{ml/min.}$$

There is thus an average pressure imbalance of about 1

mmHg and this results in a net flow of fluid out of the capillary. This volume must be accommodated in the interstitial space and cleared by (and be equal to) the lymphatic flow. However, the different parameters (especially Pt, πt and σ) used in calculating Starling's equation have been subject to marked technical variations in their measurement and there is thus a wide range of reported values.

Capillary hydrostatic and oncotic pressures

These two pressures (and in particular the πc − Pc gradient) have traditionally been the main values considered in fluid movement, largely because of their accessibility to measurement. Since the average oncotic pressure is about six times the average capillary hydrostatic pressure, it is clear that other important forces must also operate, since the lungs are wet rather than dry and since oedema can occur even when the capillary hydrostatic pressure is less than the colloid osmotic pressure.

Interstitial compliance and geometry

The compliance of the interstitial space is important in determining the consequences of fluid accumulation in the extravascular space. The interstitial pressure is normally negative, due either to lymphatic flow or the elastic recoil of the lungs or both. At these pressures, the interstitial compliance is low, so that only a small amount of extra fluid gives a considerable increase in pressure. This is because almost all of the interstitial fluid is normally in gel form, which can accommodate little extra fluid, but which is able to maintain contours without impeding diffusion. However, as further fluid enters the extravascular space, the interstitial compliance suddenly increases up to 24-fold and a large amount of fluid can now be accommodated with little further increase in interstitial pressure. This is because the fluid now accumulated is in the free or sol form and distributes according to gravity.

Fluid initially tends to collect in the thick parts of the alveolar septum, which are rich in connective tissue. The actual alveolar-capillary interface, which is the thin part of the septum, is spared so that gas exchange is not affected at this stage. The fluid subsequently migrates proximally in the perivascular and the peribronchial space and is cleared by the lymphatics. Fluid accumulation thus causes mechanical changes rather than hypoxia and it is the mechanical changes which are the chief cause of dyspnoea in pulmonary oedema.

The varying interstitial pressure/volume relation (compliance) is an important safety valve in the event of increased intravascular volume, because large amounts of fluid can pass out of the intravascular space, thus preventing increases in intravascular pressures and therefore in cardiac work.

Interstitial oncotic pressure

The interstitial albumin level (and thus oncotic pressure) is normally 50−75% of the plasma level because the pulmonary capillary is partly permeable to protein, particularly albumin. This permeability is two to four times greater than that found in peripheral tissues. Hypoalbuminaemia tends not to be a major mechanism of oedema formation, because protein is lost from the extravascular as well as the intravascular space in this condition and the oncotic pressure gradient across the capillary is relatively preserved.

Capillary permeability

A factor was incorporated into Starling's equation some 20 years after its introduction to modify the oncotic pressure gradient when it became apparent that capillaries were in fact partly permeable to protein. This factor, referred to as the capillary membrane reflection coefficient (σ), can range theoretically from 1 for membranes totally impermeable to 0 for membranes totally permeable to protein. The undamaged pulmonary capillary exhibits a value of about 0.8.

Increased pulmonary capillary permeability is thought to be a key factor in the formation of pulmonary oedema in those conditions which do not have raised intravascular pressure. This form of oedema is often referred to as a 'capillary leak syndrome'. The mechanism of pulmonary capillary damage is thought to be due to the release either locally or systemically of a variety of bioactive mediators. In Starling's equation, increased permeability implies reduced capillary membrane reflection coefficient for protein (σ) and an increased capillary filtration coefficient (Kf).

Lymphatic flow

As noted above, Starling's equation does not 'balance'. The net outward flow of fluid has to be cleared by the lymphatic flow to maintain water and solute balance. The estimated normal flow in man is about 20 ml/hour but this can be increased at least 10-fold and possibly even more when the interstitial pressure becomes positive. The lymphatic drainage is a major mechanism in keeping the lungs oedema-free.

Normal mechanisms preventing pulmonary oedema

The lungs have a significant 'safety factor' in avoiding oedema and the three main mechanisms responsible for this may be summarized as follows:
1 The lymphatic drainage has a large capacity to increase flow, especially as interstitial pressure rises to zero and above.
2 Interstitial hydrostatic pressure rises as fluid accumulates, thus decreasing the outwards hydrostatic pressure gradient.
3 Interstitial oncotic pressure falls as fluid accumulates, thus increasing the inwards oncotic pressure gradient.

As noted above, the balance of pressures does not favour keeping the lungs oedema-free, since the net positive balance results in a net outward flow of fluid. Because of this, alveolar surfaces are maintained wet rather than dry and there is a continuous flow of lymph. However, the three mechanisms protecting against oedema have an impressive reserve, so that considerable increases in capillary hydrostatic pressure or in capillary permeability can be accommodated without causing pulmonary oedema. When oedema does occur, it is not a static pathological process, but rather a part of a continuum of fluid and protein movement through the interstitium, ranging from normal flow to increased flow without change in the interstitial contents, to interstitial oedema with alveolar sparing and finally to frank alveolar flooding.

Causes of pulmonary oedema

The specific causes of pulmonary oedema may be classified as in Table 15.1. In practice the first two groups of causes are by far the most commonly encountered. It is probable that the third group, hypoalbuminaemia, is never a cause in its own right but lowers the threshold for pulmonary oedema from other causes. Groups four and five are uncommon.

Table 15.1. Causes of pulmonary oedema

Increased capillary hydrostatic pressure
  cardiogenic (left heart failure)
  blood volume overload
  pulmonary veno-occlusive disease
Increased capillary permeability
  adult respiratory distress syndrome
  viral & other pneumonia
  inhaled toxic substances
  circulating toxic agents
  disseminated intravascular coagulation
  uraemia, radiation, burns, near-drowning
Decreased plasma oncotic pressure
  hypoalbuminaemia
Decreased tissue hydrostatic pressure
  rapid lung re-expansion after pneumothorax, pleural effusion,
    pneumonectomy
Decreased lymphatic drainage
  lymphangitis carcinomatosa
  lymphangiomyomatosis
  lung transplant
Unknown mechanisms
  high altitude
  neurogenic (raised intracranial pressure)
  drug overdose (especially heroin)
  pulmonary embolism

Clinical features and diagnosis

• The *clinical features* of pulmonary oedema, regardless of cause, are dyspnoea, cough, frothy sputum and crackles on auscultation. The features of early interstitial fluid accumulation are predominantly mechanical abnormalities with decreased compliance and thus breathlessness, tachypnoea and later wheeze. More advanced fluid accumulation involving the alveolar-capillary membrane and especially with alveolar oedema gives rise to gas exchange impairment with hypoxaemia, though usually without hypercapnia or acidosis unless the process is severe. The chest X-ray shows an interstitial or alveolar infiltrate and lung function tests show hypoxaemia, hypocapnia, reduced lung volumes and decreased compliance.

• The *diagnosis* of the presence of pulmonary oedema is straightforward only in advanced stages. In early stages, its recognition is clinically difficult. Moreover, the presence of pulmonary oedema always requires the additional elucidation of the cause, because therapy is most effective when it includes specific attention to the underlying process.

In most cases, the underlying cause is apparent from the history and physical examination. Routine investigations for cardiac and systemic disease are obviously appropriate. However, when the cause is obscure or when multiple possibilities exist, the single most important investigation is the measurement of pulmonary haemodynamics using a balloon-tipped, flow-directed catheter. In particular, the measurement of the PAWP is one of the key pieces of information in making the important distinction between cardiogenic and non-cardiogenic pulmonary oedema. Cardiac output and derived haemodynamic and gas exchange indices can also be readily measured or calculated. A significantly increased PAWP (e.g. greater than 20 mmHg), especially if associated with a decreased cardiac output, indicates left heart failure in relation to circulating blood volume. A normal or low PAWP (e.g. less than 10 mmHg), especially if associated with a normal or increased cardiac output, excludes left heart failure as the cause of pulmonary oedema, provided there has been no major delay or therapeutic intervention since the diagnosis was made. Other potentially valuable measurements, such as of alveolar fluid composition or of extravascular lung water, have not yet reached the stage of ready clinical application.

Treatment

The general principles of treatment are firstly, to support the patient's disturbed gas exchange and secondly, to treat the underlying problem. Supportive treatment includes oxygenation with, in severe cases, endotracheal intubation, mechanical ventilation and positive end-expiratory pressure. Diuretic therapy with frusemide should be used unless the patient is significantly hypovolaemic and great care should be used with intravenous fluid therapy so as not to increase the cardiac filling pressures abnormally. Morphine is of symptomatic and probably physiological benefit in acute pulmonary oedema for reasons which are not entirely clear.

Specific treatment depends on the underlying disease. In pulmonary oedema of cardiogenic origin, cardiac function should be improved. Appropriate measures include inotropic therapy, sometimes with digoxin, and vasodilator therapy (e.g. nitroglycerin) to reduce preload and also afterload if the systemic vascular resistance is increased. Any concomitant arrhythmia, electrolyte imbalance, hypoxia or acidosis should also be treated. In non-cardiogenic pulmonary oedema (sometimes called low pressure pulmonary oedema or capillary leak pulmonary oedema), no specific therapy has been shown to be clinically effective, although corticosteroids in high doses are sometimes used. The best example of this form of pulmonary oedema is the adult respiratory distress syndrome and it is considered in more detail in the next chapter.

Adult Respiratory Distress Syndrome

Introduction

The adult respiratory distress syndrome (ARDS) has in recent years become the most common and the most serious respiratory complication seen in severely ill or injured patients. It has about 40 synonyms of which the most common has been shock lung.

Since its aetiology is still uncertain, it cannot be precisely defined and must therefore be described. Thus, ARDS comprises acute progressive respiratory failure occurring in patients who are already seriously ill, usually without prior pulmonary disease or present direct pulmonary damage. There is a diffuse pulmonary infiltrate on chest X-ray in the absence of increased cardiac filling pressures. There is severe hypoxaemia and the lungs are stiff. It is associated with the presence of acute pulmonary oedema due to capillary leak. The mortality is high.

Nomenclature

The specificity of ARDS as a single entity is much argued. Certainly, patients with ARDS are a heterogeneous group in that the syndrome can follow a large variety of acute disease processes. The single final end-point is more likely to be due to the limited and uniform response of the lung to different types of injury than to a single common pathogenetic mechanism in all cases. However, ARDS presents a relatively uniform pattern of clinical, physiological, pathological and radiological features and in this sense can be regarded as a single entity.

Nomenclature which permits such lumping is useful not only in communication but also in facilitating effective therapy based on a systematic physiological approach. However, some would say that ARDS is not a valid unifying term, as its use is oversimplistic and may obscure important individual entities. On balance, it would seem reasonable at present to continue to use the term ARDS while it remains useful but it is important to recognize and treat primary diseases, especially those that may have specific requirements.

Incidence

Since its first clear description in 1967, ARDS has become increasingly recognized. It has been estimated that about 600 cases per million population per year occur in industrialized societies. In addition, overt ARDS may be only the severe end of a spectrum of respiratory abnormality in seriously ill patients in that some degree of hypoxaemia can be found in most.

Aetiology and pathogenesis

Although the direct cause of ARDS is still uncertain, the likely pathogenetic mechanisms involve aggregation of formed blood elements and extensive mediator release. Granuloyctes undergo adherence, aggregation, activation and secretion following stimulation by complement (especially C5a fragment), immune complexes, peptides, PAF and leucotrienes (especially LTB4). During this process, granulocytes adhere to each other and to vascular endothelium; granulocyte aggregates then cause vascular leucostasis with resultant endothelial cell damage. Released substances include arachidonic acid metabolites (from both cyclo-oxygenase and lipo-oxygenase pathways), free oxygen radicals with toxic oxidant properties, lysosomal enzymes (particularly protease) and vasoactive substances (e.g. histamine and kinins).

Whatever the pathogenetic mechanisms involved, the final common pathway is pulmonary capillary damage with increased capillary permeability. In addition, it is likely that these effects occur at least to some extent systemically as well as in the lung.

Pathology

• *Macroscopically*, the lungs are dark, red, heavy, airless and very hard to expand. The cut surface shows haemorrhage, congestion and oedema and looks like liver. Supervening bronchopneumonia is common.
• *Microscopically*, platelet-fibrin microemboli may be seen within the first few hours but haemorrhage and oedema are the prominent findings. These are seen in the interstitium within 24−48 hours and in the alveoli within 48−72 hours, with hyaline membranes due to organized fibrin then forming. Fibrosis may occur much later.
• *Ultrastructurally*, there is endothelial damage, widened intercellular junctions and detachment of both endothelial and alveolar cells from their basement membranes.
• *Pathophysiologically*, there is increased vascular permeability with protein-rich oedema, airway closure and alveolar collapse, and pulmonary hypertension (Table 16.1). These changes give rise to defects in both gas exchange (with hypoxaemia) and lung mechanics (with decreased compliance).

Clinical features

The clinical settings of ARDS are major trauma (including burns), major surgery and serious medical illness (e.g. pancreatitis, gastrointestinal haemorrhage). Sepsis or shock appear to be common clinical antecedents. In addition, the typical patient with ARDS usually has initially or develops subsequently other associated problems, especially sepsis, shock, other organ failure or metabolic derangement.

The most common symptom is dyspnoea. There may be a dry cough initially but sputum and other features of chest

Tabel 16.1. Pathophysiology of ARDS

Change	Likely mechanisms
Pulmonary oedema	
protein-rich	Granulocyte release of:
endothelial injury	toxic oxygen radicals
increased permeability	lysosomal enzymes
	arachidonic acid metabolites
	vasoactive substances
Airway dysfunction	
airway closure	Prostanoids:
alveolar collapse	cyclo-oxygenase
increased reactivity	lipo-oxygenase
Pulmonary vascular dysfunction	
pulmonary hypertension	Thromboxan A_2
loss of hypoxic vasoconstriction	Leucotriene D_4

infection are generally later complications. On examination, there is tachypnoea and central cyanosis despite the administration of oxygen. The chest may initially appear normal but within 24−48 hours there are widespead crackles and wheezes and diminished basal breath sounds.

The clinical course of ARDS commences after a characteristic latent period of 4−24 hours between the time of the initial systemic insult and the onset of respiratory symptoms. The process tends to reach is maximum severity over the next 1−2 days. The subsequent course is very variable and although the average is 2−3 weeks, it may be as short as a few days or as long as several weeks. Acute deterioration in patients with stable or improving ARDS is common and is usually due to associated chest infection, pneumothorax or a new systemic event (particularly septicaemia).

Investigations

The most important investigations both for initial diagnosis and for subsequent management are arterial blood gas analysis and chest X-ray.
- *Arterial blood gas analysis* shows hypoxaemia, which is difficult to reverse despite an increased inspired oxygen concentration. There is thus right-to-left shunting. The arterial oxygen tension may be as low as 30−40 mmHg despite an inspired oxygen concentration of 40−60% or more. The normality or otherwise of the arterial carbon dioxide tension is determined by the ability of the patient (or the ventilator) to cope with the increased work of breathing.
- The *chest X-ray* tends to be normal initially but within 24−48 hours of the original insult there is a diffuse bilateral (though not necessarily symmetrical) pulmonary infiltrate. The early changes are those of interstitial oedema which rapidly becomes confluent and an alveolar pattern becomes apparent within the first few days. These changes have been referred to as a snowstorm appearance. This picture, though characteristic, is not specific and may be difficult to distinguish from other

diffuse infiltrative processes. By contrast with pulmonary oedema of cardiac origin, there is no cardiomegaly or pulmonary venous congestion. A typical feature of the chest X-ray of ARDS is that the appearances change only slowly with time. The chest X-ray is also important in identifying complications, such as pneumothorax, and in helping with a number of technical aspects of management, such the position of tubes and lines. Although the chest X-ray is diagnostically essential, it is not quantitative in that there is a poor correlation between the radiological changes and the clinical or functional indices of severity. Only minor radiological changes are sometimes seen, even in severe ARDS, but this is unusual and should suggest other or additional pathology, such as pulmonary embolism. The converse is more common with the chest X-ray persistently abnormal despite considerable clinical improvement, even to the point of independence from respiratory support and ambulation.

• The measurement of *cardiac filling pressures*, particularly the PAWP, is the most useful further investigation. This measurement identifies any cardiac contribution to the pulmonary oedema and also helps optimize subsequent fluid management.

Other investigations are also of importance in establishing either the diagnosis or cause of ARDS, as well as to identify underlying disease and later complications, and to guide their management.

Prevention

Since the aetiology is unknown, reliable prevention is not possible. However, it is important that the underlying acute condition predisposing to ARDS is rapidly and completely treated. Particular emphasis should be placed on early resuscitation, restoration of an adequate circulation and eradication of sepsis. A microaggregate filter should be used for blood transfusion. In high-risk patients in the first 24−48 hours, there should be careful respiratory and circulatory monitoring and alertness to the delayed respiratory deterioration that can occur some hours after apparently satisfactory resuscitation. Pharmacological measures, such as corticosteroids and aprotinin, have been used for prophylaxis and although there is some theoretical and experimental evidence to support their use, their value has not been confirmed by appropriate clinical trials.

Treatment

The mainstay of treatment of established ARDS is respiratory support with IPPV. Since there is severe right-to-left shunting, PEEP is usually required to maintain an adequate arterial oxygen tension with an acceptable inspired oxygen concentration of 60% or less. Since there also tend to be considerable mechanical abnormalities, high inflation pressures and large minute volumes are generally required to maintain adequate ventilation. Thus a relatively sophisticated ventilator is usually desirable. The combined use of IMV and CPAP (as described in Chapter 9) instead of the more traditional control mode ventilation has recently became popular in some places.

Care should be taken with fluid balance and conventional therapy is to keep the patient somewhat dehydrated provided there has been adequate resuscitation. If fluid management is difficult and especially if there is combined circulatory and/or renal dysfunction as well as respiratory failure, measurement of cardiac filling pressure is important. The use of cortico-steroids has been proposed for treatment as well as prevention and although a trial may be worthwhile in severe ARDS, this form of therapy has not been widely adopted as evidence for its efficacy is lacking. Other pharmacological agents, in-cluding cyclo-oxygenase inhibitors, oxygen radical scavengers and proline analogues, may be shown to be helpful. Although extracorporeal membrane oxygenation was shown to be not effective in a major trial, partial forms of this complex tech-nique have more recently shown promise.

Prognosis

The average mortality of patients with ARDS is about 40–60% and has remained substantially unchanged since its first des-cription in 1967. Mortality is less if there is respiratory failure alone and may be as low as 10–20% if ARDS is uncomplicated. In practice, it is commonly 70–80% because of the presence of other major problems, such as multiple organ failure or sepsis. Death is usually due to associated sepsis, cardiovascular collapse or multiple organ failure and not to respiratory failure, because the technology of respiratory support has become so effective.

The natural history of ARDS is one of gradual recovery provided the patient can be kept alive. In fact, ARDS generally undergoes complete resolution and even in patients who sustain severe disturbances of gas exchange and pulmonary mechanics, progressive return to completely normal function is usually seen over succeeding months. Occasionally, a patient will progress over several weeks to irreversible pulmonary des-truction with infection, fibrosis and even calcification. A sat-isfactory outcome is particularly dependent on the complex, expensive and prolonged efforts of a multidisciplinary health care team.

17 Lung Cancer

Introduction

Lung cancer includes a number of malignancies of which the various types of bronchogenic carcinoma are by far the most common. There has been a major increase in the prevalence and mortality of bronchogenic carcinoma in the last 50 years, so that it has been for many years by far the main cause of death from cancer in men and has recently overtaken breast cancer as the leading cause of death from cancer in women. These increases are greater than for any other form of cancer and are attributable to those forms of lung cancer which are related to tobacco smoking. There are significant differences in mortality rates in different countries but the average per 100000 population is about 150–200 in men and about 50 in women in most industrialized societies. Efforts at early detection and improved diagnostic methods have not improved the poor survival rate, which has remained substantially unchanged in recent times at only about 10% after 5 years. The high and increasing incidence of lung cancer and its low cure rate are all the more tragic when it is remembered that most cases are preventable.

Aetiology

The aetiology of bronchogenic carcinoma is considered to be related to a number of factors, including smoking, atmospheric pollution, industrial processes and genetic influences. Of these, the most important is *cigarette smoking* and there is now overwhelming evidence that it is responsible for at least 80% of cases. Changing smoking patterns within the population are responsible for the changing incidence of bronchogenic carcinoma in various groups. Smoking has became less common in men, uncommon in doctors, unchanged in teenage boys, but substantially increased in teenage girls and young women. Mortality is about 10-fold higher in smokers than in non-smokers and over 40 times higher in heavy smokers. Mortality falls in ex-smokers so that after 5 years it is 5-fold and after 15 years only twice that of non-smokers. There is a somewhat less mortality in those who do not inhale, use filtered cigarettes or smoke pipes and cigars.

Atmospheric pollution from industry and motor cars appears to play some role because mortality from bronchogenic carcinoma is higher in urban than in rural communities. This difference, however, is very much less than between smokers and non-smokers. Industrial processes involving asbestos, uranium mining, arsenic, nickel, chromate, mustard gas and possibly other substances enhance the risk of bronchogenic carcinoma, especially in smokers.

Genetic factors may possibly be relevant in view of some reported family clustering of cases and of cytogenetic abnormalities in patients compared with matched controls.

Classification

Lung cancer is classified according to its pathology into different types. These types can be so different as to represent different disorders with different manifestations and different treatment requirements. The World Health Organization classification of primary malignancies of the lung, together with the current approximate distribution of each of the different types, is as follows:

I   Squamous cell or epidermoid carcinoma (30%).
II Small cell, anaplastic ('oat cell') carcinoma (20%).
III Adenocarcinoma including bronchioloalveolar (alveolar cell) carcinoma (40%).
IV Large cell carcinoma (10%).

Combined types and unclassified neoplasms occur. Types I and II particularly, but also type III, are smoking-related. There has recently been a relative increase in the proportion of cases with type III carcinoma at the expense of type I, the previously predominant type.

The different types of lung cancer present in different ways.

• *Squamous cell carcinoma* most commonly occurs in the central airways. Though it grows relatively slowly, it may reach a large size and frequently cavitates. Metastases are frequently confined to the thorax.

• *Small cell carcinoma* also usually has a central origin. Submucosal growth often spares the overlying bronchial mucosa. Extensive lymphatic spread is usual with early and widespread metastases. Metabolic and endocrine abnormalities are common.

• *Adenocarcinoma* most commonly originates in the lung periphery. Pleural involvement is common and distinction from metastases from other sites (e.g. breast, pancreas) can be difficult without special histological techniques. Early and extensive metastases are common. Bronchioloalveolar carcinoma tends to arise peripherally and disseminate via the airways. Cancer arising in a pulmonary scar is usually an adenocarcinoma.

• *Large cell carcinoma* is also usually peripheral in origin. It is often large but otherwise behaves similarly to an adenocarcinoma.

Staging

Staging according to the extent and location of the tumour is useful for individual prognosis and for comparative purposes, especially for non-small cell cancer. The formal TNM system ('tumour', 'nodes', 'metastases') provides a grouping into four stages, namely occult, stage I (small or local tumour), stage II (local nodal metastases) and stage III (distant metastases). These criteria are detailed in Tables 17.1 and 17.2.

Clinical features

The clinical features in patients with lung cancer are very variable and are best grouped into thoracic, extrathoracic and systemic. Many patients are asymptomatic, having been detected only because of an incidental abnormality on chest X-ray.

Thoracic features

These include cough, haemoptysis, chest pain and dyspnoea. The production of large amounts of mucoid sputum is suggestive of alveolar cell (bronchioloalveolar) carcinoma. Clubbing of the fingers is common. Chest examination may show

Table 17.1. Staging classification for carcinoma of the lung

T =	*Primary tumours*
TO	No evidence of primary tumour
TX	Tumour proven by the presence of malignant cells in bronchopulmonary secretions but not visualized radiologically or bronchoscopically or any tumour that cannot be assessed
TIS	Carcinoma in situ
TI	A tumour that is 3.0 cm or less in greatest diameter, surrounded by lung or visceral pleura and without evidence of invasion proximal to a lobar bronchus at bronchoscopy. Suitable for lobectomy
T2	A tumour more than 3.0 cm in greatest diameter, or a tumour of any size which invades the visceral pleura or which has associated atelectasis or obstructive pneumonitis, extending to the hilar region; at bronchoscopy the proximal extent of demonstrable tumour must be within a lobar bronchus or at least 2.0 cm distal to the carina; any associated atelectasis or obstructive pneumonitis must involve less than an entire lung, and there must be no pleural effusion. Suitable for pneumonectomy
T3	A tumour of any size with direct extension into an adjacent structure such as the parietal pleura or chest wall, the diaphragm, or the mediastinum and its contents; or demonstrable bronchoscopically to involve a main bronchus less than 2.0 cm distal to the carina; any tumour associated with atelectasis or obstructive pneumonitis of an entire lung or pleural effusion. Not suitable for resection
N =	*Regional lymph nodes*
NO	No demonstrable metastasis to regional lymph nodes
N1	Metastasis to lymph nodes in the peribronchial or ipsilateral hilar region or both, including direct extension
N2	Metastasis to lymph nodes in the mediastinum
M =	*Distant metastasis*
MO	No distant metastasis
M1	Distant metastasis such as in scalene, supraclavicular or contralateral hilar lymph nodes, contralateral lung, brain, bones, liver, etc

Table 17.2. Stage grouping for carcinoma of the lung

Type	Definition
Occult carcinoma TX, NO, MO	An occult carcinoma with bronchopulmonary secretions containing malignant cells but without other evidence of the primary tumour or evidence of metastasis to the regional lymph nodes or distant metastasis. Site of primary tumour thus unknown
Stage I T1S, NO, MO T1, NO, MO T1, NI, MO T2, NO, MO	Carcinoma in situ A tumour that can be classified T1 without any metastasis or with metastasis to the lymph nodes in the ipsilateral hilar region only, or a tumour that can be classified T2 without any metastasis to nodes or distant metastasis. Probably resectable *Note*: TX, N1, MO and TO, N1, MO are also theoretically possible, but such a clinical diagnosis would be difficult if not impossible to make; if such a diagonsis is made, it should be included in Stage I
Stage II T2, N1 MO	A tumour classified as T2 with metastasis to the lymph nodes in the ipsilateral hilar region only. Possibly resectable
Stage III T3 with any N or M N2 with any T or M M1 with any T or N	Any tumour more extensive than T2, or any tumour with metastasis to the lymph nodes in the mediastinum, or with distant metastasis. Not resectable

signs of local obstruction with localized wheeze and rhonchi, complicating pneumonia or pleural effusion. Pneumonia associated with lung cancer typically resolves poorly. Other less common thoracic signs are listed in Table 17.3.

Extrathoracic features These are produced by metastases which may occur anywhere in the body and may be the presenting problem. The most common sites for secondary spread apart from regional lymph nodes are liver, bone and brain, followed by adrenal glands, kidneys, peritoneum and skin.

Systemic features These are often very prominent and apart from weakness and weight loss, include a number of syndromes, many of which

Table 17.3. Thoracic signs of lung cancer

Local wheeze
Pneumonia
Pleural effusion
Recurrent laryngeal or phrenic nerve involvement
Thoracic inlet (Pancoast) syndrome with:
    shoulder and arm pain
    Horner's syndrome
    brachial plexus damage
Supraclavicular lymph node involvement
Superior vena cava obstruction

are endocrine and metabolic and are caused by the release mostly of peptide hormones from the tumour. Apart from clubbing and hypertrophic pulmonary osteoarthropathy which are associated with all cell types, hypercalcaemia which is associated with squamous cell carcinoma, and carcinoid syndrome which is associated with carcinoid tumours, most of the other syndromes are chiefly associated with small cell carcinoma. The main, systemic, non-metastatic manifestations of lung cancer are listed in Table 17.4.

Diagnosis

The diagnosis is made on the basis of the chest X-ray together with cytology or histological examination of biopsy material. Asymptomatic patients may be identified from routine radiological and/or cytological examination. Symptomatic patients require formal investigation, starting with chest X-ray and bronchoscopy (with inspection, biopsy of any accessible endobronchial lesion, and brushings and washings for cytological examination). Pleural biopsy or biopsy of involved lymph nodes is sometimes diagnostic. CT scanning of the thorax, isotope or CT scanning of liver and brain and isotope scanning of bone are important staging procedures, especially if surgery is contemplated or if small cell cancer is present. Exploratory thoracotomy is sometimes required both for dia-

Table 17.4. Systemic, non-metastatic manifestations of lung cancer

General disability
  tiredness
  weakness
  anorexia
  weight loss
Connective tissue disorders
  clubbing
  hypertrophic pulmonary osteoarthropathy
  acanthosis nigricans
  dermatomyositis
Neuromuscular disorders
  myasthenia
  cerebellar degeneration
  motor and/or sensory neuropathy
  dementia
Endocrine disorders
  hypercalcaemia
  Cushing's syndrome
  syndrome of inappropriate antidiuretic hormone
  carcinoid syndrome
  hyperthyroidism
  hypoglycaemia
Haematological disorders
  thrombophlebitis
  venous thromboembolism
  non-bacterial thrombotic endocarditis
  haemolytic anaemia
  red cell aplasia
  thrombocytopenia

gnostic confirmation as well as for therapeutic purposes in the event that the lesion is operable. The diagnosis of lung cancer must be extended to both classification and staging for logical treatment.

Numerous biomarkers, produced by cancer cells or induced by their presence, have been reported as potentially useful in difficult diagnoses or in following progress. Carcinoembryonic antigen (CEA) and ectopic polypeptide hormones are the biomarkers best described to date in lung cancer.

Treatment

The treatment of lung cancer is in general most unsatisfactory. However, in individual patients, therapeutic results are sometimes good or even excellent. Without treatment, the survival is less than 1% at 3 years. Treatment modalities include surgery, radiotherapy and chemotherapy. In many cases, no specific therapy is possible or appropriate and symptomatic measures are all that can be offered.

Surgery

This offers the only hope, albeit small, of cure, so that operability is important to assess. The indication for surgery is early (stage I and II), non-small cell carcinoma. Contra-indications to surgical resection include distant metastases, mediastinal spread, small cell carcinoma, inadequate lung function and, to a lesser extent, age over 70 years. The goal of surgery is complete resection.

Lobectomy or, less commonly, pneumonectomy (or rarely segmental resection) are performed together with removal of hilar nodes. Surgeons vary in their philosophy towards the value of radical surgery in the face of more extensive invasion, e.g. involving pericardium or chest wall.The results of surgery are about 30% 5 year survival (over 50% for stage I and up to 80% for coin lesions). Survival after resection for small cell carcinoma is so poor that surgery for this is generally contra-indicated. There is an operative mortality of about 10%. Thus, since only about 25% of all cases are suitable for surgery, the average 5 year survival rate of all patients with lung cancer is about 10%.

Palliative surgery or combination with radiotherapy or chemotherapy has been disappointing. Although a variety of such combined forms of therapy have been reported and are being studied for patients with advanced disease (stage III), median survival is only a few months if there are distant metastases.

Radiotherapy

Used for localized tumour, this has been found to produce a 5 year survival of only 6%. Radical radiotherapy for inoperable carcinoma is of doubtful efficacy. Palliative radiotherapy is of value for pain, intractable cough, haemoptysis, superior vena cava obstrucion, major airway obstruction and brain metastases. Reactions to radiotherapy include oesophagitis, radiation pneumonitis and transient increase in major local obstruction, due to oedema and usually responsive to corticosteroids.

Chemotherapy

In various combination forms, this has recently been shown to produce significant temporary remission in about 50% of patients with small cell carcinoma and improvement in survival to up to 20% at 2 years. Optimal combinations of non-cross-reacting agents are continually being evaluated. New adjuvant treatment modalities are also being explored, such as autologous marrow infusion after high-dose chemotherapy, biological response modifiers (e.g. BCG vaccine) and more recently recombinant interleukin-2.

Other neoplasms of the lung

● *Primary malignant tumours* of the lung are predominantly bronchogenic carcinoma. Less common primary malignancies include mesothelioma, pulmonary lymphoma, melanoma and sarcoma. Less malignant tumours include chiefly bronchoadenoma (carcinoid tumour, cylindroma and others) and rarely papilloma, neurofibroma, haemangiopericytoma, teratoma and plasmacytoma.

● *Primary benign tumours* include chiefly hamartoma and angioma but many rare tumours (e.g. chemodectoma) have been reported.

● *Secondary (malignant) tumours* of the lung are probably more common than in other sites. The most frequent sources of the primary tumour are breast, gastrointestinal tract, urogenital system, thyroid, connective tissue sarcoma and lymphoma.

Primary benign and malignant tumours as well as metastases may also occur in intrathoracic structures other than the lung, such as mediastinum, chest wall and spine.

Pulmonary Thromboembolism

Introduction

The cardiorespiratory consequences of thromboembolism are so significant that the area is of major relevance to chest medicine. The main form of thromboembolism affecting the lungs is venous thromboembolism, i.e. venous thrombosis and pulmonary embolism. Non-embolic pulmonary thrombosis is probably quite uncommon and is generally seen only as a complication of existing severe pulmonary vascular disease (e.g. pulmonary hypertension, pulmonary vasculitis, thrombotic extension of existing pulmonary embolus).

Incidence

Whereas arterial thromboembolism is part of the epidemic of vascular disease affecting industrialized societies, venous thromboembolism is primarily a complication in hospitalized patients. Deep venous thrombosis (DVT) of the legs occurs in the calves of about 30% of hospital patients confined to bed. The incidence is much higher (60% or more) in some sub-groups of patients, particularly those having major surgery. About 20% of thrombi involving the calf extend proximally and about 10% embolize; 10−30% of pulmonary emboli are fatal. Pulmonary thromboembolism thus causes substantial morbidity and mortality in considerable numbers of hospital patients.

Pathogenesis

The underlying cause of pulmonary embolism is virtually always DVT in the legs, particularly DVT proximal to the calf. The pathogenesis of thrombosis is still well described by Virchow's triad, namely abnormalities of the vessel wall, of blood flow and of the blood itself. For venous thrombosis, the relevant components of Virchow's triad are impaired blood flow and 'hypercoagulability'. The thrombus typically commences in a valve pocket or sinus. It may have a head containing significant numbers of platelets but by far the major part of the thrombus consists of a fibrin mesh in which all the formed elements are trapped and which resembles an in vitro clot. A totally occluding thrombus forms a cast within the involved vessels. Although the majority of venous thrombi do not undergo spontaneous lysis (resolution is by organization, recanalization and collateral formation), the converse applies in pulmonary embolism where spontaneous resolution is the rule and is frequently relatively rapid. Delayed resolution occurs in patients with pulmonary hypertension or impaired fibrinolysis. Chronic thromboembolism generally represents repeated recurrence rather than persistence of the original embolism.

Clinical features

The clinical setting of pulmonary embolism is a hospital patient displaying one or more of a number of risk factors. These are age (especially over 40 years), obesity, cardiac failure, varicose veins, previous venous thromboembolism, recent major surgery (especially abdominal, orthopaedic and gynaecological), cancer, bed rest, immobilization and paralysis, and usage of the contraceptive pill. These factors are additive and several may be present in the same patient. The most potent risk factors are recent major surgery and cancer, and thus especially recent major surgery for cancer.

Most pulmonary emboli are clinically silent, which is perhaps not surprising given the huge reserve that the lungs have for filtering particulate matter. When symptoms do occur, the most frequent is dyspnoea. There may be chest pain which is usually pleuritic but sometimes central and mimicking myocardial infarction. Cough, haemoptysis and wheeze may occur.

On examination, the most common sign is tachypnoea. The temperature is frequently elevated and there may be central cyanosis. Signs in the chest may include crackles, pleural friction rub or evidence of pleural effusion. There may be features of right heart failure, including raised jugular venous pressure, loud pulmonary second sound and right ventricular gallop. A variety of arrhythmias can occur. Only the minority of patients with even extensive pulmonary embolism show clinical features of DVT of the legs.

The way in which these clinical features tend to be grouped into typical presenting patterns ranging from hyperacute to gradual is shown in Table 18.1.

Investigations

The clinical diagnosis of pulmonary embolism is unreliable. Not only are most pulmonary emboli silent but those clinical features which are commonly seen are all non-specific. However, these features are important as they raise clinical suspicion and lead to appropriate investigation (Table 18.2).
• A *chest X-ray* should always be performed. Although even in major pulmonary embolism it is frequently completely nor-

Table 18.1. Patterns of clinical presentation of pulmonary embolism

Collapse
Acute hypotension
Acute right ventricular failure
Pulmonary hypertension
Dysponea or tachypnoea alone
Pneumonitis (incomplete infarct)
Pulmonary infarction

Table 18.2. Investigation of pulmonary embolism	Chest X-ray
	ECG
	Arterial blood gas analysis
	Biochemical/haematological tests
	Lung scanning
	Pulmonary angiography

mal, it may show suggestive features, such as infarction (areas of consolidation), diaphragmatic elevation, pleural effusion, proximal pulmonary artery distension and focal oligaemia. More importantly, the chest X-ray excludes other possible differential diagnoses, such as pneumothorax, pneumonia and cardiac failure.

• An *ECG* should also be performed routinely. Although it is abnormal in over 80% of cases of major embolism, the specific features of acute cor pulmonale are apparent in only about 25%. These include an S wave in lead 1, Q wave in lead 3 and inverted T wave in lead 3 (S1, Q3, T3), right axis deviation, right atrial hypertrophy and right bundle branch block. More commonly, only non-specific ST-T changes are seen or a variety of arrhythmias. However, like the chest X-ray, the ECG helps exclude other potential differential diagnoses, such as myocardial infarction.

• *Arterial blood gas analysis* is commonly performed, though its complications outweigh its value should subsequent anticoagulant or thrombolytic therapy be given. Typically, the arterial oxygen tension is reduced. The arterial carbon dioxide tension is also reduced, reflecting hyperventilation. The arterial pH is raised and bicarbonate normal, reflecting the acuteness of the process. These arterial blood gas values are entirely non-specific and are similar to those seen in a variety of other acute respiratory problems, including asthma, pneumonia and pulmonary oedema. However, normal blood gas values make the diagnosis of major pulmonary embolism less likely.

• A variety of *biochemical tests* have in the past been proposed as diagnostically helpful in pulmonary embolism. However, the classical triad of a raised lactic dehydrogenase (LDH) and bilirubin but normal aspartate aminotransferase (AST) has been found to occur in only about 4% of cases of even major embolism. The only laboratory measurement of any value is the serum level of fibrin degradation products (FDPs). Provided disseminated intravascular coagulation can be excluded, raised levels of FDPs are suggestive of pulmonary embolism.

• The two definitive diagnostic techniques are lung scanning and pulmonary angiography. *Lung scanning* is generally the most useful test both for diagnosis and for follow-up. Its results correlate well with pulmonary angiography and with post-mortem findings. Its chief strength is that false negative results are rare (i.e. it is very sensitive). However, the presence of perfusion defects on lung scan is non-specific, although

specificity is increased if a concomitant chest X-ray and preferably ventilation lung scan are normal. The lung scan cannot
actually diagnose pulmonary embolism but can only assess its
probability. The probability is increased with the size of the
perfusion defect, the presence of multiple defects and a venti-
lation/blood flow mismatch. Although the lung scan in many
patients shows a sufficiently high or low probability of pulmonary embolism to permit reliable clinical management, a
variable proportion of lung scans (ranging from 15–40% of
cases) shows a medium probability and thus cannot advance
the diagnosis.

• *Pulmonary angiography* is the diagnostic yardstick during
life. However, it is complex and invasive and much less widely
used than lung scanning. The procedure is, however, safe
even in very sick patients and permits haemodynamic measurements as well as angiography. The specific criterion for dia-
gnosing an embolus is the demonstration of an intralumenal
filling defect with a sharp cut-off (thus the thrombus is actually
'seen'). However, there are a number of technical and clinical
pitfalls in angiographic diagnosis and in addition an incomplete
study may be not clearly interpretable.

A strategy for the appropriate use of diagnostic investigations is shown in Table 18.3.

Table 18.3 Strategy for diagnosis of pulmonary embolism

Test	Result	Diagnosis	Action
Perfusion lung scan	Normal	No PE	No treatment
	Abnormal	?	Pulmonary angiogram or ventilation lung scan
Ventilation (+ perfusion) lung scan	Low probability	No PE	No treatment
	High probability	PE	Treatment
	Medium probability	?	Pulmonary angiogram or empirical treatment or venogram of legs for DVT*

PE = pulmonary embolism.
*Venography does not clarify the diagnosis of PE itself but, as DVT is usual with PE and as treatment with
anticoagulants is similar in both DVT and PE, venography will generally assist in making a correct decision
regarding treatment in suspected PE.

Prevention

It has been said that pulmonary embolism demonstrates a
unique triad in clinical medicine, in that it is a common condition with a significant mortality but difficult diagnosis. Thus,
the key to its solution lies in prevention. Its effective prevention requires that the high-risk patient can be identified
and that suitable prophylactic measures are available. These
requirements can nowadays be met. The high-risk patient is
identifiable as outlined above. Proven prophylactic measures
available for use in such patients include low dose heparin,

dextran, oral anticoagulants and methods to increase venous blood flow in the legs. Of these measures, the use of low dose heparin (5000 units twice daily) is the most generally appropriate. Both venous thrombosis and non-fatal and fatal pulmonary embolism are reduced by about 60% by low dose heparin.

Treatment

The treatment of established pulmonary embolism depends both on its extent and the underlying illness of the patient. Supportive treatment including oxygen and analgesia is required if the patient is symptomatic. Vasoactive drug infusion such as with isoprenaline is indicated for hypotension. Anticoagulant therapy with full doses of heparin is indicated in all cases, unless there is a life-threatening bleeding complication. Thrombolytic therapy, usually with streptokinase, has been shown to enhance dramatically the lysis of major emboli. Surgical embolectomy is nowadays performed only infrequently, since the advent of both effective prevention and of medical (enzymic) embolectomy. Inferior vena cava interruption is indicated for embolism that is recurrent despite adequate anticoagulant therapy.

Prognosis

Pulmonary embolism is still the commonest cause of death in hospital, being responsible for probably about 10% of all deaths and contributing to about 25%. Careful post-mortem examination has been reported to show the presence of some degree of pulmonary embolism in over 50% of patients.

The outlook in pulmonary embolism is as follows. The acute mortality is probably about 20%. Three quarters of these deaths occur within the first 2 hours of the event. About 70% of pulmonary emboli are clinically unrecognized. About 30% are clinically recognized but of these only about 5% have massive and 5% major embolism. Thus, only about 10% of patients with pulmonary embolism have the so-called classical features permitting ready clinical recognition. Importantly, probably as many patients as are clinically recognized are erroneously thought to have pulmonary embolism and are thus exposed to the risks of treatment without the benefits. Of those patients who had pulmonary embolism but were unrecognized, probably half recur. With treatment, however, the incidence of recurrence is low and usually falls to background level in about 6 weeks. Similarly, the mortality of patients on adequate anticoagulant therapy is extremely low.

The Lung in Systemic Disease

Introduction

Since most disease processes affect at least to some extent multiple sites in the body, their classification based on main organ abnormalities may be convenient but can be somewhat arbitrary. Thus, for the lung, generalized diseases such as sarcoidosis or even major infections such as tuberculosis are usually discussed as pulmonary disorders, even though their implications are in fact widespread. Even pulmonary oedema of direct cardiac origin is considered a lung problem because its chief clinical consequences are respiratory. On the other hand, many systemic diseases or diseases of other organs have implications for the lung which, while not prominent enough to consider as specific pulmonary problems, are nevertheless clinically significant. These diseases are considered in this chapter.

Collagen-vascular diseases (connective tissue disorders)

Systemic lupus erythematosus (SLE)

This is a multi-system disease of unknown aetiology and variable course. It affects the lung in a primary manner in about 50% of cases. Pulmonary involvement includes direct lupus pneumonitis (with fever, cough, dyspnoea and patchy radiological opacities) or more commonly, the secondary pulmonary infections of the compromised host. Diffuse interstitial fibrosis may rarely occur. Pleural effusion or pleurisy is probably the commonest pulmonary manifestation. Myopathy may affect the diaphragm, with resultant dyspnoea and basal atelectasis. The lung may also be secondarily affected because of lupus involvement of the heart or kidneys. In general, the pulmonary manifestations parallel the course of the underlying disease, which is steroid-responsive and usually has a fairly good long-term prognosis.

Systemic sclerosis (scleroderma)

This is a sclerosing condition of unknown aetiology involving the connective tissue of many organs. The lungs are clinically involved in about 40% of cases and pathologically (at autopsy) in about 90%. The most common pulmonary changes are diffuse interstitial fibrosis, especially in the lower zones, which may not be radiologically apparent even when dyspnoea is present. There may be associated vascular lesions but pleural involvement is uncommon. There is an increased incidence of lung cancer, especially of the alveolar cell type. The lung may also be secondarily affected because of scleroderma involvement of the heart, kidneys, oesophagus (with resultant aspiration) or chest wall and diaphragm. Corticosteroid therapy is not usually effective and the average survival is only a few years.

Dermatomyositis and/or polymyositis

This may sometimes be associated with pulmonary fibrosis. Aspiration due to pharyngeal muscle weakness may occur and there is an increased incidence of lung cancer. Corticosteroids appear to be of help.

Mixed connective tissue disease

This is associated with pulmonary fibrosis in most cases.

Other types of systemic disease involving the lung

Rheumatoid arthritis

This may be associated with a number of pulmonary manifestations. These include pleurisy and pleural effusions in particular, but also diffuse fibrosing alveolitis, lung nodules and pneumoconiosis (Caplan's syndrome). 'Rheumatoid lung' as manifested by an abnormal chest X-ray and reduced gas transfer, together with one of the above processes, occurs in about 40% of patients with rheumatoid arthritis. It is responsive to corticosteroids in some cases. Other less common changes include obliterative bronchiolitis, pulmonary vasculitis and rheumatoid pharyngitis. There is an increased incidence of respiratory infections.

Sjögren's syndrome

This is commonly considered a variant of rheumatoid disease and can occur in association with any of the connective tissue disorders. Lung involvement is similar to that seen in rheumatoid arthritis.

Ankylosing spondylitis

This is associated with an unusual form of pulmonary fibrosis affecting chiefly the upper zones.

Polyarteritis nodosa (PAN)

This is a rare disease characterized by necrotizing vasculitis. Lung involvement occurs in about a third of patients and is associated with eosinophilia. PAN appears to merge at one end into the benign forms of PIE and at the other into Wegener's granulomatosis. The form of pulmonary involvement associated with asthma is sometimes called *Churg—Strauss syndrome* (allergic granulomatosis and vasculitis). Treatment with corticosteroids is indicated.

Behçet's syndrome

This comprises relapsing iridocyclitis with recurrent oral, genital and skin ulceration. It is due to an underlying vasculitis and may occasionally cause diffuse transient pulmonary infiltrates. Pulmonary embolism may be involved in this process.

Relapsing polychondritis	This is a rare disease which may involve the cartilage of the pharynx and trachea with resultant major airway obstruction.
Stevens—Johnson syndrome (erythema multiforme)	This is a diffuse vasculitis provoked by a number of drugs, especially sulphonamides, and causing widespread skin lesions. Diffuse or localized lung shadows may occur.
Tuberous sclerosis	This affects many organs, especially the CNS, and may be associated with diffuse pulmonary fibrosis in some cases.
Neurofibromatosis (von Recklinghausen's disease)	This may be associated with either diffuse pulmonary fibrosis or multiple intrathoracic tumours, including mediastinal neuro-fibromas.
Lipid storage diseases	Lipid storage diseases of each of the ten known types (e.g. Gaucher's disease) are characterized by accumulaton of different lipids in various tissues, including pulmonary infiltration.
Renal failure	This has a number of associations with lung disease. These particularly include acute glomerulonephritis in some bacterial infections, Goodpasture's syndrome, Wegener's granulomatosis, collagen-vascular or connective tissue disorders, disseminated intravascular coagulation (DIC), some drug reactions and transplant complications. Uraemia is associated with pleurisy and pleural effusion, often as part of a polyserositis and associated with a pulmonary oedema-like picture ('uraemic lung'). Respiratory problems may also occur during dialysis, e.g. pleural effusion during peritoneal dialysis and hypoxaemia (probably due to leucoagglutination and complement activation) during haemodialysis.
Neurological diseases	Disorders such as motor neurone disease and dysautonomia (usually of the familial type) interfere with pharyngeal and oesophageal function and may lead to aspiration pneumonitis.
Obesity	This may cause respiratory failure but the mechanisms are not as well understood as might be thought. Obesity leads to decreased lung volumes, decreased lung and chest wall compliance, areas of low ventilation/perfusion ratios and obstructive sleep apnoea. There may sometimes be a reduced respiratory drive. There is then hypoxaemia, hypercapnia, polycythaemia, cor pulmonale and somnolence (Pickwickian syndrome). Weight reduction may dramatically improve the clinical situation and prognosis.

Pulmonary hypertension   Anatomical variations
Sleep apnoea syndromes   Pleural diseases
Cystic fibrosis   Mediastinal diseases
Bronchiectasis   Chest wall diseases
Obliterative bronchiolitis   Diaphragmatic diseases
Tracheopathia osteoplastica

Pulmonary hypertension

Pulmonary hypertension is a common association of many lung diseases. It also follows a number of non-pulmonary, especially cardiac, disorders. Pulmonary hypertension is defined as an increase in the pulmonary artery pressure above 30/15 mmHg.

Cor pulmonale is right ventricular hypertrophy and/or dilatation secondary to pulmonary disease and in response to pulmonary hypertension. There may or may not be overt right ventricular failure. The development of right ventricular hypertrophy implies that the process is chronic. Right ventricular dilatation, however, may be acute.

The causes of pulmonary hypertension are:
- *Increased left atrial pressure* due to left heart failure. This causes passive pulmonary hypertension. Since the pulmonary venous pressure is increased, pulmonary oedema eventually occurs.
- *Increased pulmonary blood flow* due to left-to-right shunt. This causes hyperkinetic pulmonary hypertension.
- *Increased pulmonary vascular resistance*. This may be due to vascular constriction, obliteration or obstruction. Vasoconstriction is usually due to hypoxia, obliteration to diffuse parenchymal damage, vasculitis or rarely veno-occlusive disease, and obstruction to pulmonary embolism or thrombosis.

Regardless of the initial cause, secondary structural changes eventually occur in the pulmonary arteries. In addition, reactive vasoconstriction occurs in some patients. Both of these complications further exacerbate the hypertension.

In practice, the main cause of pulmonary hypertension is parenchymal damage resulting from chronic airways obstruction, particularly chronic bronchitis. Other important causes include diffuse interstitial lung disease, bronchiectasis, kyphoscoliosis, vasculitis, primary pulmonary hypertension and pulmonary veno-occulsive disease. However, any lung disease if sufficiently severe and widespread can cause pulmonary hypertension.

The clinical features include symptoms due to low cardiac output, such as fatigue, dyspnoea and angina. Physical examination shows a variety of cardiac findings, including right ventricular hypertrophy, loud pulmonary component of the second sound, right heart gallop and in advanced cases, systolic ejection click and pulmonary diastolic and tricuspid pansystolic murmurs. There may be evidence of overt right ventricular failure with increased jugular venous pressure and prominent 'a' wave, hepatomegaly and peripheral oedema.

The investigation of patients with pulmonary hypertension requires chest X-ray, ECG and appropriate lung function tests. In addition, right heart catheterization is indicated to (a) confirm the presence of pulmonary hypertension, (b) indicate the left atrial pressure (indirectly by the PAWP), (c) demonstrate the presence of left-to-right shunt by right heart blood-gas sampling, (d) permit calculation of pulmonary vascular resistance, and (e) allow pulmonary angiography.

The treatment of pulmonary hypertension and cor pulmonale is that of the underlying condition. Diuretics and especially digitalis should be used with considerable caution. In appropriate cases, long-term oxygen therapy is helpful.

● *Primary pulmonary hypertension* is an uncommon condition of unknown aetiology primarily affecting young women. Its distinction from chronic, recurrent, pulmonary thrombo-embolism is not always possible. The chief symptoms are fatigue, dyspnoea and syncope on exertion. Physical signs of cor pulmonale are usually marked, often with peripheral vasoconstriction and cyanosis. There is no effective therapy and the average survival is only about 3 years from the onset of symptoms.

Sleep apnoea syndromes

Sleep may be associated with disordered breathing in the sudden infant death syndrome (SIDS), Pickwickian syndrome and sleep apnoea syndromes. In addition, periodic breathing (including Cheyne–Stokes breathing) is seen during sleep in patients with chronic pulmonary, cardiac or CNS disease and in some normal subjects, for example at altitude.

● *Central sleep apnoea* may occur in rapid eye movement (REM) or non-REM sleep. In the former, breathing is independent of metabolic stimuli, except for hypoxia, so that apnoea is brief, unless there is loss of chemoreceptor sensitivity to hypoxia. In the latter, breathing is dependent on metabolic controls, so that prolonged apnoea occurs if the normal controls are inoperative due to brain stem or chemoreceptor damage.

● *Obstructive sleep apnoea* results from upper airway obstruction, sometimes due to definable anatomical or pathological lesions but sometimes without clinically apparent abnormalities. This form of apnoea occurs during both REM and non-REM sleep. The precise mechanism leading to upper airway obstruction is unclear. There is probably a relaxation of pharyngeal muscle tone during REM sleep but with persistent diaphragmatic activity and thus upper airway narrowing and closure. There may also be impairment of mucosal sensory activity. The distinction between central and obstructive sleep apnoea syndromes, however, is not sharp since both types commonly occur together. Moreover, central aponea may be triggered by upper airway closure via an inspiratory inhibitory reflex.

• Patients with chronic airways obstruction may suffer exacerbation during sleep, with hypoventilation during non-REM sleep and apnoea during REM sleep. These patients also suffer from nocturnal depression of cough and mucociliary clearance and consequent sputum accumulation.

Patients with sleep apnoea syndromes (or their partners) complain of various sleep disorders including snoring, nightmares, morning headache, daytime somnolence and sometimes chronic insomnia. Most patients are middle-aged men, are often overweight and have normal lung function when alert during the daytime. They usually have obstructive sleep apnoea due to upper airway obstruction. Serious cardiac arrhythmias, including heart block, asystole and ventricular tachycardia can occur during the episodes of nocturnal apnoea. Patients with chronic airways obstruction and sleep apnoea suffer not only marked acute exacerbations of hypoxaemia, hypercapnia and pulmonary hypertension during the episodes themselves but also chronic deterioration, especially of cor pulmonale.

While a confident diagnosis of sleep apnoea can usually be made from descriptions given by a sleeping partner, formal studies in a laboratory with measurement during sleep of ventilation, repiratory movements, eye movements and gas exchange (polysomnography) will confirm the type of apnoea and quantify the degree of respiratory failure. Treatment measures include weight loss, avoidance of nocturnal sedation including alcohol, neck support with a surgical collar, CPAP applied with a nasal mask, nocturnal oxygen therapy, sometimes uvulopalatopharyngoplasty and occasionally permanent tracheostomy.

Cystic fibrosis

Cystic fibrosis is a common genetic disorder transmitted as an autosomal recessive trait. It is a generalized disorder that affects exocrine glands so that their secretions are abnormally viscid. The nature of the underlying biochemical defect is unclear. The pulmonary changes are secondary to bronchial obstruction from viscid secretions with secondary infection, atelectasis, fibrosis and bronchiectasis.

Clinical features include cough, sputum, dyspnoea and wheeze. Physical examination shows cyanosis, clubbing, hyperinflation and signs of cor pulmonale. The diagnosis is made on the basis of increased sodium and chloride levels in sweat (greater than 60 mmol/l in children and 80 mmol/l in adults).

Treatment is with physiotherapy (postural drainage and breathing exercises), nebulized mist therapy, bronchodilators and intensive antibiotic therapy. Pancreatic enzyme replacement is required, as is adequate salt and water balance. With these recent improvements in treatment, patients with cystic fibrosis are now surviving into adulthood.

Bronchiectasis

Bronchiectasis is defined on anatomical grounds as chronic abnormal dilatation of larger bronchi. The prevalence of bronchiectasis has decreased greatly in advanced societies in recent times since potent antibiotic therapy became available for severe, necrotizing lung infections. Its aetiology probably includes congenital factors as well as severe respiratory infection with airway obstruction and damage due to chronic inflammation. The pooling of bronchial secretions rich in inflammatory products and intracellular proteases contributes to ongoing weakening of the bronchial wall. The association of congenital dextrocardia, bronchiectasis and sinusitis is referred to as *Kartagener's syndrome*. Bronchiectasis may complicate cystic fibrosis, hypogammaglobulinaemia, rheumatoid lung and asthmatic pulmonary eosinophilia.

The clinical features are cough and purulent sputum. The sputum can be copious and particularly offensive. Haemoptysis, dyspnoea and wheeze may occur. Physical examination reveals clubbing of the fingers and crackles on auscultation.

The diagnosis is made by bronchography (or autopsy). The bronchographic distinction between cylindrical, fusiform and saccular changes probably has little clinical sgnificance. Treatment is primarily with physiotherapy and antibiotics, the latter preferably only for exacerbations in most patients. Surgical resection is only occasionally indicated nowadays. Prevention is of major importance and includes particularly the prompt and effective treatment of respiratory infections and of obstruction by foreign bodies.

Obliterative bronchiolitis

Obliterative bronchiolitis (bronchiolitis fibrosa obliterans) is a rare condition and probably a very severe form of chronic bronchitis with pathological changes implied by its name. It is most usually due to the inhalation a few weeks previously of toxic gases, for example industrial chemicals such as nitrogen dioxide or military poisons. It has occasionally followed severe infections. The chest X-ray shows diffuse fine nodules with subsequent hyperinflation. The prognosis is considered poor.

Tracheopathia osteoplastica

Tracheopathia osteoplastica (bronchopathia osteoplastica) is a rare disease with cartilagenous and sometimes calcified plaques projecting into the lumen of the major airways. The plaques originate from the tracheal cartilages. Most patients are older men and the process is asymptomatic, though there may be resultant airways obstruction.

Anatomical variations

Anatomical variations may occur in the airways and lung, as elsewhere in the body.

Congenital tracheal atresia and some forms of stenosis are associated with tracheo-oesophageal fistula.

Abnormal patterns of bronchial branching may occur, including right-to-left reversal which is usually associated with situs inversus.

Tracheal diverticula, bronchial cysts and congenital bronchiectasis may occur.

Agenesis (absence) or hypoplasia of a lung or lobe is usually associated with other congenital anomalies elsewhere.

Bronchopulmonary sequestration refers to an area of lung without bronchial connection and with an aberrant and systemic blood supply. It is one of the more common and important abnormalities.

Extra or absent fissures are common but of little clinical siginficance.

Abnormalities of the pulmonary circulation may include arteriovenous fistulae, distal pulmonary artery stenosis and anomalous venous return.

Other congenital conditions are familial and have been already referred to elsewhere, namely cystic fibrosis, Kartagener's syndrome, α_1-antitryspin deficiency, immunological disorders, tuberous sclerosis and neurofibromatosis. Congenital anomalies may also occur of mediastinum (e.g. cysts), diaphragm (e.g. eventration, hernia) or chest wall (e.g. pectus excavatum or carinatum).

Pleural diseases

● *Pneumothorax* implies the presence of air within the pleural cavity and is associated with concomitant reduction in lung expansion. The condition usually develops suddenly. While it may be associated with mild symptoms and an insignificant degree of lung collapse, more usually the sudden onset of breathlessness and pleuritic pain heralds a pneumothorax of significant size which demands treatment. A pneumothorax may steadily increase in size producing compression of the ipsilateral lung and eventually causing displacement of the mediastinum, compression of the contralateral lung and circulatory embarrassment. Immediate treatment of this tension pneumothorax is required.

The physical signs of pneumothorax may be quite subtle unless the pneumothorax is large. Reduced chest expansion, hyper-resonant percussion note and diminished intensity of breath sounds on the affected side should be sought. Striking a coin applied to the chest wall with another coin will produce a ringing sound on auscultation over the area (coin percussion of Trousseau). Cardiac displacement away from the affected side, tachycardia, hypotension and general chest hyperinflation are signs of tension pneumothorax. A chest X-ray is essential to confirm the presence of a pneumothorax and to assess its size and likely cause.

Pneumothorax can arise spontaneously either in otherwise healthy subjects (primary pneumothorax) or as a complication of another lung disorder (secondary pneumothorax). Traumatic pneumothorax can follow direct injury to the thoracic cage or pulmonary barotrauma associated with mechanical ventilation (Table 20.1). Young tall males who are otherwise healthy appear to be at most risk of spontaneous pneumothorax. This is thought to be due to the greater apical distending forces operating in association with elastic recoil (which declines with age) and the pleural pressure gradient which is proportional to vertical lung height. There may be also some

Table 20.1. Causes and
classification of
pneumothorax

Spontaneous
Primary:
  young tall males
  catamenial
Secondary:
  asthma, obstructive bronchitis
  emphysema
  interstitial lung disease
  Marfan's syndrome

Traumatic
Open:
  penetrating chest wall injury
Closed:
  chest wall injury
  pulmonary barotrauma
  transbronchial lung biopsy
  subclavian venous cannulation

Tension
  complicating any type of pneumothorax

inherent weakness in the subpleural apical tissue, such as small blebs.

Treatment of pneumothorax depends on its size and cause. Traumatic pneumothorax is best treated with insertion of an intercostal catheter and underwater seal since, in addition, there is often blood in the pleural cavity (haemopneumothorax). A small spontaneous pneumothorax (about 25% reduction of lung volume or less) may be managed conservatively but larger pneumothoraces require either direct aspiration or intercostal catheter insertion. Resolution of a small pneumothorax normally requires 5–7 days but this can be substantially hastened by administering oxygen, which promotes reabsorption by exaggerating the diffusion gradient for nitrogen between the blood and intrathoracic gas.

There is a risk of ipsilateral recurrence of about 25% within 2 years. Pleurodesis is usually performed after one or two recurrences and thoracotomy may be required for a persisting bronchopleural fistula. Review of patients with apparent primary spontaneous pneumothorax is essential to exclude underlying pathology requiring treatment.

• *Pleurisy* or inflammation of the parietal pleura is always due to underlying pulmonary disease. It is associated with chest pain, often severe, and with a pleural friction rub on auscultation. Dry or fibrinous pleurisy may be followed later by pleural effusion.

• *Pleural effusion* may be either a transudate or exudate (less than or greater than 30 g/l protein, respectively) or contain blood (haemothorax), pus (empyema) or chyle (chylothorax). An effusion must contain at least 500 ml before it can be detected clinically and 100–300 ml before it is apparent radiologically. The mechanisms of fluid production are salt, water and protein imbalance (e.g. congestive cardiac failure), increased capillary pressure (e.g. left ventricular failure), increased capillary permeability (e.g. inflammation) or decreased lymphatic drainage (e.g. neoplasm). The first two mechanisms give rise to transudates and the latter two to exudates. A transudate is sometimes called a hydrothorax. The pleural effusion may lie free in the pleural space or be loculated either in the general space or into lobular or subpulmonary spaces.

The chief causes of pleural effusions are congestive cardiac failure (transudates) and bacterial pneumonia, pulmonary infarction and secondary malignancy (exudates)(see Chapter 21). Haemothorax and empyema have been previously described in relation to the underlying conditions which give rise to them. Chylothorax is due to obstruction or disruption of the thoracic duct or right lymphatic duct by tumour, surgery or trauma.

The chief investigation is pleural aspiration (with or without pleural biopsy). The fluid is examined for macroscopic appearance, biochemistry including protein, glucose and LDH, cytology including differential white cell count and microbiology including microscopy and culture (Table 20.2).

• *Pleural tumours* may occasionally be primary and include fibroma (localized mesothelioma) and diffuse malignant mesothelioma. The former is treated by surgical resection; no effective treatment is available for the latter.

Mediastinal diseases

Mediastinal diseases include chiefly cysts and tumours. There are many different types of lesions and their nature depends greatly on their site within the mediastinum (Table 20.3, Fig. 20.1). The most common, in order, are neurogenic tumours (especially neurofibroma), cysts (especially bronchogenic or

Table 20.2. Examination of pleural fluid

Macroscopic appearance
straw-coloured (transudate, exudate)
purulent (empyema)
blood-stained (haemothorax)
milky (chylothorax)

Biochemistry
protein   < 30 g/l transudate
           > 30 g/l exudate
glucose   N ≈ 50% plasma level
           decreased in:
              tuberculosis
              malignancy
              rheumatoid disease
              post-pneumonic
              empyema
LDH   increased in:
              inflammation

Cytology

Microbiology

Table 20.3. Types of mediastinal lesions

Superior
  thymoma
  teratoma
  lymphoma
  retrosternal thyroid
  cystic hygroma
  aortic aneurysm
  haemangioma
  abscess
  lymphadenopathy
  oesophageal lesion
Anterior
  thymoma
  teratoma
  lymphoma
  retrosternal thyroid
  pericardial or pleuropericardial cyst
  cystic hygroma
  hernia through foramen of Morgagni
Middle
  aortic aneurysm or other great vessel abnormality
  bronchogenic cyst
  lipoma
  cardiac tumour
Posterior
  neurogenic tumour (neurofibroma)
  gastro-oesophageal or bronchogenic cyst
  oesophageal lesion
  meningocele
  aortic aneurysm
  hernia through foramen of Bochdalek

pericardial), thymoma (more often benign than malignant), teratoma (also more often benign than malignant), lymphoma and retrosternal thyroid.

• *Acute mediastinitis* usually follows oesophageal perforation or rupture. It requires appropriate antibiotic therapy and surgical drainage of any abscess.

• *Chronic mediastinitis* is usually associated with a progressive fibrotic process. The cause is unknown but it may be related to other fibrosing diseases, especially retroperitoneal fibrosis but also Riedel's thyroiditis, Dupuytren's contracture, Peyronie's disease and sclerosing cholangitis. Methysergide therapy for migraine has been implicated in some cases. Sometimes the disease is localized (e.g. to the hilar region). There is no effective therapy.

The clinical features of mediastinal disease may include pain, dysphagia, hoarseness, stridor, cough, haemoptysis and dyspnoea. Physical examination may reveal Horner's syndrome, superior vena cave obstruction, enlarged cervical lymph nodes or pleural effusion. Investigations include chest X-ray, often including tomography or aortography, CT scanning and sometimes bronchoscopy and mediastinoscopy.

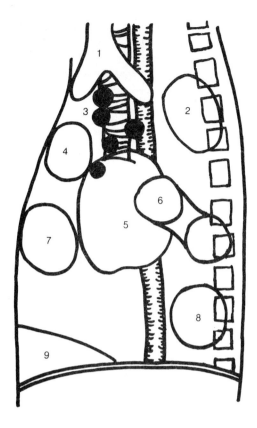

Fig. 20.1. Lateral representation of the mediastinum showing typical sites of common space-occupying lesions. (1) Thyroid. (2) Neurofibroma. (3) Lymph nodes. (4) Thymus. (5) Lipoma. (6) Foregut anomalies. (7) Teratoma. (8) Meningocele. (9) Pleuropericardial cyst. (Modified from Crofton & Douglas, 1981).

Chest wall diseases

Chest wall diseases include congenital abnormalities, trauma, inflammatory lesions and tumours. Congenital abnormalities have been referred to above (see Anatomical variations) and trauma previously (see Chapter 14). Inflammatory lesions are uncommon but may include most acute and chronic thoracic infections. A specific inflammatory condition is *Tietze's syndrome* (costochondritis) which is characterized by pain and swelling over the upper costal cartilages. The cause is unknown, the chest X-ray normal and gradual remission the rule. *Coarctation of the aorta* causes notching of the inferior borders of the ribs, especially the 4th to 8th. *Tumours* may be primary or secondary, usually the latter. Most primary tumours are benign.

Kyphoscoliosis results in pulmonary distortion due to the chest wall deformity, with decreased lung volumes in some parts of the lung and compensatory hyperinflation in others. Overall, there is a mixed obstructive and restrictive defect with hypoxaemia, recurrent chest infections and cor pulmonale in advanced cases.

Diaphragmatic diseases Diaphragmatic diseases include eventration, hernia, paralysis, spasmodic disorders (hiccup, tonic spasm, flutter), trichiniasis, trauma, subdiaphragmatic abscess and rare tumours.

Eventration refers to elevation and paradoxical movement of one hemidiaphragm, usually the left. It is commonly congenital.

Paralysis of one or rarely both hemidiaphragms occurs with lesions of the phrenic nerve. Such lesions result from tumours, trauma or neurological disorders. Orthopnoea and paradoxical movement of the diaphragm in relation to the chest wall during inspiration are typical clinical features of diaphragmatic paralysis.

Practical Outline of Some Specific Respiratory Problems

Dyspnoea	Solitary lung nodule
Wheeze	Lung cavitation
Haemoptysis	Diffuse pulmonary infiltrate
Pleural effusion	

There are a number of specific respiratory problems, either symptoms or findings, for which elucidation is particularly helped by having a check-list of causes or investigations. These problems include the symptoms of dyspnoea, wheeze and haemoptysis, and the radiological findings of pleural effusion, solitary lung nodule, lung cavitation and diffuse pulmonary infiltrate.

Dyspnoea

The chief causes of dyspnoea are listed in Table 21.1, together with their major distinguishing features. The term dyspnoea is used here in its broadest sense and also includes some sensations which might more strictly be called hyperpnoea. A vast number of conditions may at times be associated with dyspnoea and Table 21.1 lists only those causes which are relatively common and in which dyspnoea is a prominent symptom.

It is worth noting that there are three causes of dyspnoea which are associated typically with normal physical examination and chest X-ray (provided non-pulmonary conditions, such as anaemia, have been excluded). These are pulmonary embolism, early interstitial lung disease and psychogenic dyspnoea. Most other causes of dyspnoea have typical clinical or radiological features.

One of the common difficulties in elucidating the origin of dysponea is the distinction between respiratory and cardiac causes, particularly if disorders of both are present together. In most cases, a careful history and physical examination with simple cardiac and respiratory tests, including chest X-ray, ECG, spirometry and arterial blood-gas analysis, will clarify the issue satisfactorily. Some patients with wheeze may have either bronchial asthma or cardiac asthma, and broncho-provocation studies can be of specific diagnostic value. In patients with significant, combined respiratory and cardiac disease, it may be impossible to be confident of the cause of dyspnoea without further investigation, particularly exercise testing.

Wheeze

The ten chief causes of wheeze are listed in Table 21.2 in their approximate order of importance. It is important to remember that local obstructive lesions in the trachea may produce

Table 21.1. Chief causes of dyspnoea

	Major distinguishing features				
	History	Physical examination	Chest X-ray	Lung function tests	Other
Pulmonary					
asthma	*	*	—	*	—
chronic bronchitis and emphysema	*	*	†	*	—
pulmonary oedema	*	*	†	—	—
pulmonary embolism	†	—	—	†	scan, angiogram
cancer	—	—	*	—	histology
interstitial disease	—	†	†	*	histology
collagen-vascular disease	*	*	*	†	serology, histology
hypersensitivity pneumonitis	*	*	*	*	serology
PIE	*	*	*	—	haematology
acute lung irritation	*	*	*	—	—
Cardiac					
left ventricular failure	*	*	*	—	*
mitral valve disease	*	*	*	—	*
constrictive pericarditis	*	*	*	—	*
Systemic					
anaemia	*	*	—	—	Hb
metabolic acidosis	*	—	—	—	pH
neurological lesions	*	*	—	—	—
psychogenic	†	—	—	—	—

* indicates that the feature, usually in combination with others, is sufficiently characteristic to be diagnostic. † indicates that the feature is variable and may even sometimes be normal. — indicates that the feature is usually non-contributory to diagnosis and may be normal.

either stridor or a diffusely audible wheeze. Apart from pulmonary embolism and sometimes asthma and chronic bronchitis, all the other causes of wheeze are associated with an abnormal chest X-ray. Also, except for pulmonary embolism, the more common conditions are generally apparent from their clinical features.

Table 21.2. Chief causes of wheeze

Asthma
Chronic bronchitis and emphysema
Pulmonary oedema
Pulmonary embolism
Aspiration pneumonitis
Drug reaction
Acute lung irritation
Cystic fibrosis
PIE
Polyarteritis nodosa

Exclude: stridor (= laryngeal obstruction), local wheeze (= local obstruction).

| Haemoptysis | The ten chief causes of haemoptysis are listed in Table 21.3 in their approximate order of importance. Although the cause may be apparent from the clinical features and/or chest X-ray, bronchoscopy is usually required to clarify the diagnosis. Even after extensive investigation, some episodes of haemoptysis are not satisfactorily explained. |

Table 21.3. Chief causes of haemoptysis

Acute chest infection
  (bronchitis, pneumonia)
Carcinoma
  (also rarely bronchial adenoma)
Chronic bronchitis
Pulmonary infarction
Acute pulmonary oedema
  (left ventricular failure)
Foreign body
Bronchiectasis, lung abscess
Tuberculosis
Systemic bleeding disorder
Pulmonary vasculitis

Pleural effusion

The chief causes of the five types of pleural effusion are listed in Table 21.4. The underlying diagnosis is based on clinical features, chest X-ray and examination of aspirated pleural fluid.

Solitary lung nodule

The seven chief causes of a solitary lung nodule are listed in Table 21.5 in their approximate order of importance. The diagnosis is not usually able to be made from the clinical features, most patients being asymptomatic. It frequently requires comparison with previous films (if available), tomography, CT scanning, bronchoscopy and sometimes thoracotomy and resection.

Lung cavitation

The seven chief causes of one or more lung cavities are listed in Table 21.6 in their approximate order of importance. This ranking varies greatly and is influenced by many factors, such as age, smoking habits, socioeconomic status and occupation. While the diagnosis may be aided by the clinical features, it generally requires at least bronchoscopy and cytological and microbiological examination of bronchial secretions, washings and brushings.

Diffuse pulmonary infiltrate

The most common of a very large number of causes of diffuse pulmonary infiltration are listed in Table 21.7 in very approximate order of importance. The number of causes is so large that no single diagnostic approach will cover them all. Much help can be gained from the clinical setting and clinical features. Diagnosis is usually additionally dependent on bronchoscopy, microbiological and cytological examination of washings and brushings, and sometimes biopsy.

Table 21.4. Chief causes of pleural effusion

Transudate
congestive cardiac failure
hypoproteinaemia
Meig's syndrome
polyserositis
peritoneal dialysis
Exudate
bacterial pneumonia
pulmonary infarction
malignancy (metastases)
tuberculosis
subphrenic abscess
pancreatitis
collagen-vascular disease
lymphoma
uraemia
Empyema
bacterial pneumonia
subphrenic abscess
penetrating injury
Haemothorax
trauma
malignancy
pulmonary infarction
leukaemia
tuberculosis
'bloody tap'
Chylothorax
malignancy
trauma
surgery

The most common causes in each group are printed in bold type

Table 21.5. Chief causes of a solitary lung nodule

Bronchogenic carcinoma
Metastatic carcinoma
Benign tumour
Pulmonary infarct
Lung abscess
Tuberculosis
Hydatid cyst

Table 21.6. Chief cause of one or more lung cavities

Bronchogenic carcinoma
Necrotizing pneumonia
Lung abscess
Tuberculosis
Infected cyst or bulla
Rheumatoid lung
Wegener's granulomatosis

Table 21.7. Chief causes of a diffuse pulmonary infiltrate

Pneumonia
Interstitial lung disease
    (sarcoidosis, diffuse fibrosing alveolitis, other interstitial lung
    disease, collagen-vascular disease, PIE)
Malignancy
    (lymphoma, metastases, lymphangitis carcinomatosa)
Pulmonary oedema
Adult respiratory distress syndrome
Pneumoconiosis
Hypersensitivity pneumonitis
Aspiration pneumonitis
Drug reaction
Wegener's granulomatosis
Goodpasture's syndrome
Miliary tuberculosis
Radiation pneumonitis
Uraemia

Further Reading

The following is a list of classic publications and recent reviews suggested for further reading.

General references

Baum G.L. & Wolinsky E. (1983) *Textbook of Pulmonary Diseases*, 3rd edn. Little, Brown & Co., Boston.

Cherniack R.M. (ed.)(1986) *Current Therapy of Respiratory Disease*, 2nd edn. W.B. Saunders Co., Philadelphia.

Crofton J. & Douglas A. (1981) *Respiratory Diseases*, 3rd edn. Blackwell Scientific Publications, Oxford.

Dunnill M.S. (1982) *Pulmonary Pathology*. Churchill Livingstone, Edinburgh.

Flenley D.C. & Petty T.L. (eds.)(1982) *Recent Advances in Respiratory Medicine*, 3rd edn. Churchill Livingstone, Edinburgh.

George R.B., Light R.W. & Matthay R.A. (eds.)(1983) *Chest Medicine*. Churchill Livingstone, Edinburgh.

Hinshaw H.C. & Murray J.F. (1980) *Diseases of the Chest*. W.B. Saunders Co., Philadelphia.

Matthay R.A., Matthay M.A. & Wiedemann H.P. (eds.)(1986) *Annual Review of Pulmonary and Critical Care Medicine*. Hanley & Belfus, Philadelphia.

Murray J.F. (1986) *The Normal Lung*. W.B. Saunders Co., Philadelphia.

Phelan P.D., Landau L.I. & Olinsky A. (1982) *Respiratory Illness in Children*, 2nd edn. Blackwell Scientific Publications, Oxford.

Robin E.D. (1983−6) Respiratory medicine. In *Scientific American Medicine*, Section 14 (eds. Rubenstein E. & Federman D.D.). Scientific American, New York.

Sahn S.A. (1982) *Pulmonary Emergencies*. Churchill Livingstone, Edinburgh.

Sonne L. (1983) *Key References in Pulmonary Disorders*. Churchill Livingstone, Edinburgh.

Weinberger S. (1986) *Principles of Pulmonary Medicine*. W.B. Saunders Co., Philadelphia.

Specific topics

Chapter 1   Structure of the Respiratory System

Nagaishi C. (1972) *Functional Anatomy and Histology of the Lung*. University Park Press, Baltimore.

Weibel E.R. (1973) Morphological basis of alveolar capillary gas exchange. *Physiol Rev*, **53**, 413−495.

Chapter 2 Respiratory Physiology

Cade, J.F. (1984) Respiration. In *Clinical Physiology*, 3rd edn., pp. 96−153 (eds. Campbell E.J.M., Dickinson C.J., Slater J.D.H., Edwards C.R.W. & Sikora K.). Blackwell Scientific Publications, Oxford.

Fishman, A.P. (ed.)(1986) The respiratory system. In *Handbook of Physiology*, Section 3. American Physiological Society, Bethesda.

Hedley-Whyte J., Burgess G.E., Feeley T.W. & Miller M.G. (1976) *Applied Physiology of Respiratory Care*. Little, Brown & Co. Boston.

Phillipson E.A. (1978) Control of breathing during sleep. *Am Rev Respir Dis*, **118**, 909−939.

Wagner P.D. (1977) Diffusion and chemical reactions in pulmonary gas exchange. *Physiol Rev*, **57**, 257−312.

West J.B. (1977) Ventilation-perfusion relationships. *Am Rev Respir Dis*, **116**, 919−943.

—— (1985a) *Respiratory Physiology*, 3rd edn. Williams & Wilkins, Baltimore.

—— (1985b) *Ventilation/Blood Flow and Gas Exchange*, 4th edn. Blackwell Scientific Publications, Oxford.

Chapter 3 Respiratory Symptoms and Signs

Burrows. B. (1975) Pulmonary terms and symbols. A report of the ACCP-ATS Joint Committee on pulmonary nomenclature. *Chest*, **67**, 583−593.

Forgacs P. (1978) The functional basis of pulmonary sounds. *Chest*, **73**, 399−405.

Kraman S.S. (ed.)(1985) Lung sounds. *Semin Resp Med*, **6** (3).

Chapter 4 Lung Function Tests

Bates, D.V., Macklem P.T. & Christie R.V. (1971) *Respiratory Function in Disease*, 2nd edn. W.B. Saunders Co., Philadelphia.

Cade, J.F. (1984) Respiration. In *Clinical Physiology*, 3rd edn., pp. 96−153 (eds. Campbell E.J.M., Dickinson C.J., Slater J.D.H., Edwards C.R.W. & Sikora K.). Blackwell Scientific Publications, Oxford.

Cherniack R.M. (ed.)(1983) Pulmonary function testing. *Semin Resp Med*, **4** (3).

Comroe J.H., Forster R.E., Dubois, A.B., Briscoe W.A. & Carlsen E. (1962) *The Lung*, 2nd edn. Year Book Medical Publishers, Chicago.

Cotes J.E. (1975) *Lung Function: Assessment and Application in Medicine*, 3rd edn. Blackwell Scientific Publications, Oxford.

Jones N.L. & Campbell E.J.M. (1982) *Clinical Exercise Testing*. W.B. Saunders Co., Philadelphia.

West J.B. (1982) *Pulmonary Pathophysiology*. Williams & Wilkins, Baltimore.

Chapter 5 Imaging, Bronchoscopy and Other Investigations

Brown L.R. & Muhm J.R. (1983) Computed tomography of the thorax. *Chest*, **83**, 806−813.

Clark T.J.H. (ed.)(1981) *Clinical Investigation of Respiratory Disease*. Chapman & Hall, London.

Crystal R.G., Reynolds H.Y. & Kalica A.R. (1986) Bronchoalveolar lavage. *Chest*, **90**, 122−131.

McLoud T.C. (ed.)(1984) Chest radiology. *Clin Chest Med*, **5** (2).
Putman C. (ed.)(1983) Lung imaging. *Semin Resp Med*, **5** (1).
Robin E.D. & Burke C.M. (1986) Routine chest X-ray examination. *Chest*, **90**, 258–262.
Sanderson D.R. (ed.)(1981) Diagnostic techniques. *Semin Resp Med*, **3** (1).

Chapter 6   Blood Gas Analysis

Jones N.L. (1980) *Blood Gases and Acid-Base Physiology*. Brian C. Decker, New York.
Sutton J.R. & Jones N.L. (eds.)(1981) Hypoxia and acid-base interaction. *Semin Resp Med*, **3** (2).

Chapter 7   Respiratory Failure

Campbell E.J.M. (1965) Respiratory failure. *Br Med J*, **1**, 1451–1460.
Pontoppidan H., Geffin B. & Lowenstein E. (1972) Acute respiratory failure in the adult. *N Engl J Med*, **287**, 690–698, 743–752, 799–806.

Chapter 8   Respiratory Therapy

Kirby R.R., Smith R.A. & Desautels D.A. (eds.)(1985) *Mechanical Ventilation*. Churchill Livingstone, Edinburgh.
MacDonnell K.F. & Segal M.S. (eds.)(1977) *Current Respiratory Care*. Little, Brown & Co., Boston.
O'Donohue W.J. (ed.)(1984) *Current Advances in Respiratory Care*. American College of Chest Physicians, Park Ridge.
Petty T.L. (1982) *Intensive and Rehabilitative Respiratory Care*, 3rd edn. Lea & Febiger, Philadelphia.
Zagelbaum G.L. & Pare J.A.P. (1982) *Manual of Acute Respiratory Care*. Little, Brown & Co., Boston.

Chapter 9   Immumology and the Lung

Chapel H. & Haeney M. (1984) *Essentials of Clinical Immunology*. Blackwell Scientific Publications, Oxford.
Clancy R.L. (1986) The respiratory tract. In *Clinical Immunology Illustrated*, Chapter 11 (eds. Wells J.V. & Nelson D.S.). Williams & Wilkins, Sydney.
David J. (1979–86) Immunology. In *Scientific American Medicine*, Section 6 (eds. Rubinstein E. & Federman D.D.). Scientific American, New York.
Salvaggio J.E. & Stankus R.F. (eds.) (1983) Immune factors in pulmonary disease. *Clin Chest Med*, **4** (1).
—— & deShazo R.D. (eds.) (1984) Immunologic lung disease. *Semin Resp Med*, **5** (3).

Chapter 10   Asthma

Bailey W.C. (ed.)(1984) Asthma. *Clin Chest Med*, **5** (4).
Clark T.J.H. & Godfrey S. (1983) *Asthma*. Chapman & Hall, London.
—— & Rees J. (1985) *Practical Management of Asthma*. Martin Dunitz, London.
Gershwin M.E. (ed.)(1986) *Bronchial Asthma*. Grune & Stratton, New York.
Hargreave F.E. & Woolcock A.J. (eds.)(1985) *Airway Responsiveness — Measurement and Interpretation*. Astra, Mississauga.

Hodgkin J.E. (ed.)(1986) International scope of asthma. *Chest*, **90**, (suppl.) 5.

O'Byrne P.M. (1986) Airway inflammation and airway hyper-responsiveness. *Chest*, **90**, 575−577.

Rebuck A.S. & Read J. (1971) Assessment and management of severe asthma. *Am J Med*, **51**, 788−798.

Schulman E.S. (1986) The role of mast cell derived mediators in airway hyper-responsiveness. *Chest*, **90**, 578−583.

Sheppard D. (1986) Mechanisms of bronchoconstriction from non-immunologic environmental stimuli. *Chest*, **90**, 584−587.

Weiss E.B. (1985) *Bronchial Asthma*. Little, Brown & Co., Boston.

Williams M.H. (ed.)(1980) Asthma and airway reactivity. *Semin Resp Med*, **1** (4).

Chapter 11   Chronic Bronchitis and Emphysema

Berend N. (1983) Small airways disease. *Aust NZ J Med*, **13**, 393−397.

Cohen A.B. (ed.)(1986) Current and future therapy for chronic obstructive pulmonary diseases. *Semin Resp Med*, **8** (2).

Flenley D.C. (1985) Long term home oxygen therapy. *Chest*, **87**, 99−103.

Fletcher C.M., Peto R., Trinker C. & Speizer F. (1976) *The Natural History of Chronic Bronchitis and Emphysema*. Oxford University Press, Oxford.

Montenegro H.D. (1984) *Chronic Obstructive Pulmonary Disease*. Churchill Livingstone, Edinburgh.

Petty T.L. (1982) *Prescribing Home Oxygen for COPD*. Thieme-Stratton, New York.

—— (ed.)(1985) *Chronic Obstructive Pulmonary Disease*. Marcel Dekker, New York.

Snider G.L. (ed.)(1983) Emphysema. *Clin Chest Med*, **4** (3).

Chapter 12   Respiratory Infections

Huber G.L. (ed.)(1980) Respiratory tract defenses. *Semin Resp Med*, **1** (3).

Reynolds H.Y. (ed.)(1981) Pulmonary infections. *Clin Chest Med*, **2** (1).

Simon H.B. & Schwartz M.N. (1985) Pulmonary infections. In *Scientific American Medicine*, Section 7 (eds. Rubinstein E. & Federman D.D.). Scientific American, New York.

Stamm A.M. & Dismukes W.E. (1983) Current therapy of pulmonary and disseminated fungal diseases. *Chest*, **83**, 911−917.

Chapter 13   Interstitial Lung Disease

Fulmer J.D. (1982) The interstitial lung diseases. *Chest*, **82**, 172−178.

—— (ed.)(1982) Interstitial lung diseases. *Clin Chest Med*, **3** (3).

James D.G. (ed.)(1986) Sarcoidosis of the respiratory system. *Semin Resp Med*, **8** (1).

Turner-Warwick M. (ed.)(1984) Interstitial lung disease. *Semin Resp Med*, **6** (1).

Chapter 14   Other Pulmonary Insults

Brooks S.M. (ed.)(1986) Occuptional lung disease. *Semin Resp Med*, **7** (3).

——, Lockey J.E. & Harber P. (eds.)(1981) Occupational lung diseases. *Clin Chest Med*, **2** (2, 3).

Daughtry D.C. (ed.)(1980) *Thoracic Trauma*. Little, Brown & Co., Boston.

Gee J.B.L. (ed.)(1984) *Occupational Lung Disease*. Churchill Livingstone, Edinburgh.

Jackson R.M. (1985) Pulmonary oxygen toxicity. *Chest*, **88**, 900–905.

Modell J.H. (1971) *The Pathophysiology and Treatment of Drowning and Near-Drowning*. Thomas, Springfield.

Morgan W.K.C. & Seaton A. (1975) *Occupational Lung Diseases*. W.B. Saunders Co., Philadelphia.

Parkes W.R. (1982) *Occupational Lung Disorders*, 2nd edn. Butterworth, London.

Rosenow E.C. (ed.)(1980) Drug-induced lung diseases. *Semin Resp Med*, **2** (2).

Rubinstein E. (1986) Water-related accidents. In *Scientific American Medicine*, Section 8 (eds. Rubinstein E. & Federman D.D.). Scientific American, New York.

Chapter 15   Pulmonary Oedema

Brigham K.L. (ed.)(1983) Pulmonary edema. *Semin Resp Med*, **4**, (4).

Civetta J.M. (1979) A new look at the Starling equation. *Crit Care Med*, **7**, 84–91.

Matthay M.A. (ed.)(1985) Pulmonary edema. *Clin Chest Med*, **6** (3).

Robin E.D., Cross C.E. & Zelis R. (1973) Pulmonary edema. *N Engl J Med*, **288**, 239–246, 292–304.

Staub N.C. (1974) Pulmonary oedema. *Physiol Rev*, **54**, 678–811.

Chapter 16   Adult Respiratory Distress Syndrome

Andreadis N.A. & Petty T.L. (eds.)(1986) New basic and clinical science in adult respiratory distress syndrome. *Semin Resp Med* (suppl.).

Ashbaugh D.G., Bigelow D.B., Petty T.L. & Levine B.E. (1967) Acute respiratory distress in adults. *Lancet*, **2** 319–323.

Bone R.C. (ed.)(1982) Adult respiratory distress syndrome. *Clin Chest Med*, **3** (1).

Kazemi H., Hyman A.L. & Kadowitz P.J. (eds.)(1986) *Acute Lung Injury*. PSG, Littleton.

Chapter 17   Lung Cancer

Carr D.T. (ed.)(1982) Cancer of the lung. *Semin Resp Med*, **3** (3), **4** (1).

Matthay R.A. (ed.)(1982) Recent advances in lung cancer. *Clin Chest Med*, **3** (2).

Skarin A.T. (1986) Respiratory cancer. In *Scientific American Medicine*, Section 12 (eds. Rubinstein E. & Federman D.D.). Scientific American, New York.

Chapter 18   Pulmonary Thromboembolism

Colman R.W., Hirsh J., Marder V.J. & Salzman E.W. (eds.) (1982) *Hemostasis and Thrombosis*. Lippincott, Philadelphia.

Hume M., Sevitt S. & Thomas D.P. (1970) *Venous Thrombosis and Pulmonary Embolism*. Harvard University Press, Cambridge.

Heyers T.M. (ed.)(1984) Pulmonary embolism and hypertension. *Clin Chest Med*, **5** (3).

Rubinstein E. (1986) Thromboembolism. In *Scientific American Medicine*, Section 1 (eds. Rubinstein E. & Federman D.D.). Scientific American, New York.

Sasahara A.A. & Stein M. (eds.)(1965) *Pulmonary Embolic Disease*. Grune & Stratton, New York.

——, Sonnenblick E.H. & Lesch M. (eds.)(1975) *Pulmonary Emboli*. Grune & Stratton, New York.

Chapter 19   The Lung in Systemic Disease

See general references

Chapter 20 Miscellaneous Pulmonary Disorders

Davis P.B. (ed.)(1985) Cystic fibrosis. *Semin Resp Med*, **6** (4).

Fletcher E.C. (ed.)(1986) *Abnormalities of Respiration during Sleep*. Grune & Stratton, New York.

Ingbar D. & Gee J.B. (1985) Pathophysiology and treatment of sleep apnea. *Annu Rev Med*, **36**, 369–395.

Kryger M.H. (ed.)(1985) Sleep disorders. *Clin Chest Med*, **6** (4).

Light R.W. (ed.)(1985) Pleural diseases. *Clin Chest Med*, **6** (1).

Robin E.D. (1983) Pulmonary vascular disease and cor pulmonale. In *Scientific American Medicine*, Section 1 (eds. Rubinstein E. & Federman D.D.). Scientific American, New York.

Tobin M.J., Cohn M.A. & Sackner M.A. (1983) Breathing abnormalities during sleep. *Arch Intern Med*, **143**, 1221–1228.

Voelkel N.F. (1985) Pulmonary hypertension and pulmonary vascular disease. *Semin Resp Med*, **7** (2).

Weinberger S.E., Weiss S.T., Cohen W.R., Woodrow Weiss J. & Johnson T.S. (1980) Pregnancy and the lung. *Amer Rev Respir Dis*, **121**, 559–581.

Index